I Don't Know
WHY I ACT LIKE THIS

How to Uncover the Relationship between Your Mental Health and Your Emotions

Carrie Vanderbilt

ISBN: 9798847872881

REVIEWS

Reviews and feedback help improve this book and the author. If you enjoy this book, we would greatly appreciate it if you could take a few moments to share your opinion and post a review on Amazon.

Download The Audio Version of This Book for Free! If you love listening to audiobooks on-the-go or enjoy the narration as you read along I have great news for you. You can download this book for **FREE** just by signing up for a FREE 30-day audible trial. Just use the links below

FOR AUDIBLE UK: **FOR AUDIBLE US:**

CONTENTS

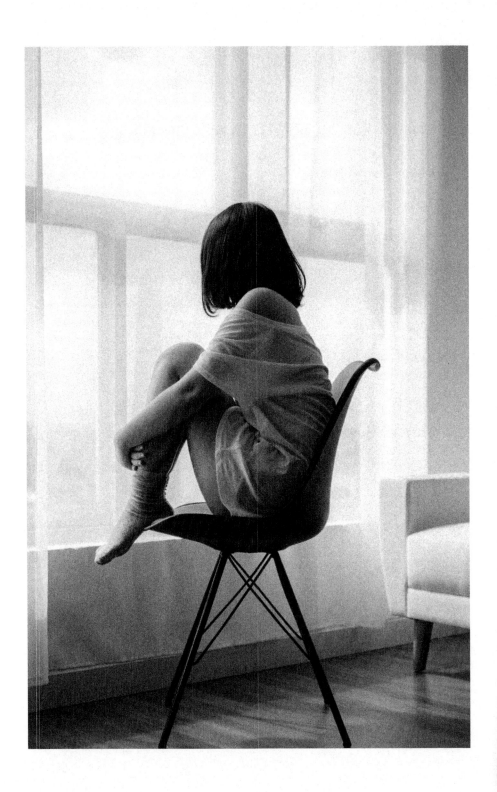

INTRODUCTION

How are you feeling today?

If that sounds like a loaded question, it's meant to be. How any of us "feel" at any given time is rarely captured in a single word, and like images in a kaleidoscope, our emotional, mental, and physical state can flip flop in an instant, taking us from a friendly, comfortable state of mind to one that is strange, unfamiliar, and scary.

So, keeping in mind that this is a loaded question, I'll ask again: How are you feeling today?

For many of us, the answer is not one word. It may be a full sentence, paragraph, or even a chapter. Emotions are rarely one-dimensional and are inspired by everything that touches our existence.

Have you ever flown into a rage because your sleeve caught on a door handle? Have you ever found yourself sobbing uncontrollably because the meal you made came out slightly less than perfect? Or are you prone to lying awake all night, mentally racing through a terrible highlight reel of all the times you were awkward or failed? And furthermore, have you ever been ashamed, embarrassed, or flat out angry at yourself for having this seemingly unprovoked reaction to something trivial and out of your control?

Emotions allow us to experience the world around us from a unique perspective that often defies logic, cultural norms, and even our own good sense. When we're experiencing something passionately, we're often grateful for whatever strange combination of neural impulses and chemicals that enable us to "feel" this way. On the other hand, when we're toiling in the aftermath of a tragic event, we often wish all those feelings would just go away.

That's because emotions are– simply put– extremely complicated. You might be feeling sad but hopeful but also disgusted and a little hungry all at once. One of my favorite and frequently referenced movie quotes from JK Rowlings' *Harry Potter and the Order of the Phoenix*. I feel this passage sums up how complicated emotions can be and nails it when it comes to the phenomenon that is human emotion:

> *"Well, obviously, she's feeling very sad, because of Cedric dying. Then I expect she's feeling confused because she liked Cedric and now, she likes Harry, and she can't work out who she likes best. Then she'll be feeling guilty, thinking it's an insult to Cedric's memory to be kissing Harry at all, and she'll be worrying about what everyone else might say about her if she starts going out with Harry. And she probably can't work out what her feelings towards Harry are anyway, because he was the one who was with Cedric when Cedric died, so that's all very mixed up and painful. Oh, and she's afraid she's going to be thrown off the Ravenclaw Quidditch team because she's flying so badly."*

A slightly stunned silence greeted the end of this speech, then Ron said, "One person can't feel all that at once, they'd explode."

— *J.K. Rowling, Harry Potter and the Order of the Phoenix*

Chances are high that you have the ability to identify with the complex cobweb of multiple emotions referenced in this passage. You're feeling this way because of that stimulus, and this way because of this other thing and feeling both feelings at once creates its own layer of response... to the point where we often get completely lost in what we're feeling and why.

The biological processes of emotions are still not entirely known. Science is working to understand how this three-pound wad of electric Jell-O that resides in our skull can have so much influence and control over our well-being, but much of the human brain remains a mystery. We know that our memories and experiences impact our emotional response to various stimuli. The trauma that we experience throughout our life tends to throw another lens on the kaleidoscope of our emotions, as does the way we manage to cope with that trauma.

Then we must consider our overall mental health. Much like emotions, our mental health can wax and wane. A good day can turn sour quickly, while a dreary day has a sliver of potential of turning itself around if all the stars align. According to studies conducted in 2020 by the National Institute of Mental Health (NIMH), one out of five adults in the United States lives with some type of mental health issue. To do some quick math, that's approximately 52.9 million individuals who are experiencing some type of atypical mental function. To explore that number from another lens, that's 21% of the population.

The definition the NIMH provides for "any mental illness" is a broad explanation for what these people experience:

Any mental illness (AMI) is defined as a mental, behavioral, or emotional disorder. AMI can vary in impact, ranging from no impairment to mild, moderate, and even severe impairment

So, what does this all mean in the context of this book? It means that even if you are not currently living with mental health issues, it is extremely likely that someone close to you is.

Furthermore, it also means that you or someone close to you may be struggling with mental health issues at any given time. That may mean feeling lousy, tired, sad, invalidated, useless, hopeless, drained, unmotivated, overwhelmed, disconnected, confused, on edge, fearful, worried, agitated, angry, enraged, violent, foolish, awkward, embarrassed, and/or panicked, often on a rolling basis.

Due to whatever mysterious process interprets the chemical and electrical impulses in our brain and body to make us "feel" different things, mental and emotional health are closely linked. And since both can change quickly and without much warning, it often seems to those of us who are impacted by mental illness that living day to day can be much like living on a raft castaway at sea. On some days, it may seem that we're just one heavy wave of feeling away from capsizing, while other days, our emotional seascape is as smooth as glass.

This book is not going to cure your mental illness. It will not solve all your perceived emotional "problems," nor does it take the place of professional mental health assistance. I'm not a doctor, and your therapist probably hasn't heard of this book yet, as it's just one of the many, many tools available for those who are struggling with connecting their head, mind, and heart.

I was initially diagnosed with mental health issues in the early 1990s. While that doesn't seem too long ago, it was an entirely different landscape for those who "weren't quite right," as we politely whispered to each other. Mental illness was still a stigmatized topic. I remember sitting across from my father at our favorite Chinese restaurant. Being the 1990s, there were mirrors everywhere, and the dining room was super dim. I blurted out to my father that I thought I might need to see a therapist before going away to college, and I immediately scanned the room, looking to see who had overheard me airing my shame so publicly. No one heard– no one could have, given the seating arrangement of large plush booths– but his loudly hissed "We'll talk about this later" still resonates as one of the most shameful moments in my history of dealing with mental illness.

In fact, getting a diagnosis and treatment felt like a mysterious journey through darkness. I was asked a series of questions by a doctor, then told I had depression and to take these pills. When I reported back that the pills were inspiring some wicked hallucinations, I was told to take half a pill. When that didn't quell the giant visage of Tom Selleck following me along the highway, I was told to take half a pill every other day. I quit taking pills altogether and didn't bother seeking help for my mental health for another ten years. Why bother? It was all clearly in my head.

By the time I re-emerged into thinking that maybe I should try getting professional help again, I had developed terrible coping mechanisms. I had ostracized most of the people I thought I loved. I had been living out of my car for a few months. I was an angry and terrified wad of loosely cobbled together coping mechanisms, most of which entailed always being defensive. But at this point, I was fairly convinced that I was going to drop dead at any time, thanks to the hypochondria that had been left unchecked for over twenty years.

This book is for people like me. Like I was, before I decided that I wanted to have some sort of say in how I felt at any given time. Like I am now, self-aware but not always ready to engage in my own self-preservation. Like I hope to be some day, confident and eager to see what each new day brings.

My goal is to present to each reader a journey through their current mental and emotional health and provide exercises that I have personally used and learned from my mentors in the mental health community. Consider me a sympathetic, empathetic, and sometimes just pathetic tour guide through this journey. I'm a real person who has real problems and is working through them.

I know that some of you will read this and think that it is complete hooey. There are days when I think it's just a bunch of junk, too. One of the many oddly fascinating things about having mental health issues is that occasionally, you decide you don't want, need, or especially deserve help. When you're in one of these mind frames, it's really easy to dismiss any practical application of assistance, no matter how small or well-intended.

Furthermore, not every type of exercise or assistance works for everyone. There will be many types of exercise in the following chapters from mindfulness and awareness tools to activities that make you explore your inner thought process or acknowledge your emotions. This may not be the right time in your mental health journey to complete these exercises, so please do not feel that you are required to complete each exercise as we go along. Think of them as tools and keep them in your toolbox in an easy-to-find place, so you know exactly where to find them when your mind and emotions need a little mending.

I ask that you keep an open mind and consider the points made in this book. Not every approach to mental health works for every individual. There are things in here that might trigger you, upset you, or send you into an overthinking spiral. It all depends on how you're feeling on any given day, right? Please know that I am never coming from a place of attack, but of collaboration. I will make every attempt to openly communicate any potential triggers as well as provide guidance towards reframing any negative thoughts that are conjured up by the exercises I share. In return, I ask that you read with an open mind and proceed cautiously when you're having those raw, tender-feeling days.

I'd like to mention again that this book is not intended to replace or provide any type of professional medical assistance. My goal is not to be your long-distance therapist, but to be another companion in the march against the tempest that mental illness can be. Together, we'll learn how to connect with your emotions. Once you know the beasts you face, you'll be able to choose the right tools from your toolbox to help you quell them. We'll investigate how each trigger and emotional response can impact our well-being as well as our relationships with others.

I wish I could say that this book will solve all your problems. I also wish I could say that all my problems have been solved. Unfortunately, that's not how this battle works. There is no magic word or perfect potion that prevents us from having to work towards equilibrium in our mental health. It's a constant uphill battle, and though there are often restful plateaus, the road is often steep and perilous. The exercises included in this book may be hard to complete at times, and other times seem almost ridiculously easy. You will likely cycle through a variety of emotions when considering how difficult working on mental health can be.

But the fact that you want to try is the most important part of this equation. You might not be ready to dive head-first into mental and emotional reframing— in fact, that might be beyond the scope of most of our healing processes. However, if you're willing to dip in a single toe, then maybe another, we can take baby steps together towards connecting with even our most confusing emotions.

THE "WHO AND WHAT" OF MENTAL AND EMOTIONAL HEALTH

Our understanding, appreciation, and expression of our mental and emotional health can be a muddy swamp to wade through. Sometimes, it can be difficult to tell if what we're experiencing is an emotional outburst due to our mental health or mental illness symptoms that are being exacerbated by our current emotional state.

> *Example:*
> *Sally has been diagnosed with PTSD. She saw an advertisement that didn't necessarily trigger her, but it made her feel some different emotions. The more she dwelled on these emotions, the more she thought about the ad, which made her feel increasingly uncomfortable. After a few hours, she finds herself completely overwhelmed by feelings of despair and sadness. She starts relating her feelings to the hopelessness she felt after her traumatic episode, and eventually, she is completely triggered.*

Is this an emotional outburst, or part of living with PTSD? Can you identify a time when you found yourself feeling more emotional than others perceived the situation warranted?

When emotions run high, it can be even harder to sort out what you're feeling, what has triggered you, and why you're feeling this way. That means you may have already acted on your emotions before you could clearly think through the situation.

For many of us, it may seem that there's no difference. Sometimes, you just feel a certain way. Some diagnoses, such as generalized anxiety disorder and clinical depression, represent the most prevalent emotion exhibited by patients.

But, as many people who cope with GAD or depression share, that's not the only emotion or expression of their condition. So, what's the difference between mental illness and emotional problems?

Mental Health and Mood

In the medical community, the term "mental health" is used to describe an individual's cognitive ability– that is, how they receive, interpret, store, and respond to information. Emotional health, on the other hand, specifically targets the emotional response one has to information, especially information that can be stressful.

But what is and isn't "stressful" to any individual is up to debate. Some of us can staunchly chomp popcorn while watching a slasher film, while others become overwhelmed by simple tasks. For many of us, these wildly varied reactions can happen simultaneously or in rapid succession, which adds to the mystery of mental illness and emotional disorders. Sometimes we take certain incidents in stride, while others can cause us a significant amount of stress.

We've all heard that a certain level of stress is healthy. In fact, many experts believe that our survival instincts are based on maintaining a certain level of stress that aids in our perception of potential danger. But for those of us who live with mental illnesses, what is and is not stressful can be based around our current mental status as well as triggers caused by past trauma.

Example: It's just been one of those mornings. You woke up late, you stepped in whatever mess your pet made during the night, and you ran out of toothpaste. You discovered a stain on the outfit you were going to wear, and of course it's laundry day, so you had to cobble together something that may or may not even match. Then you couldn't find your car keys, and just as you were leaving the house, your jacket sleeve got caught on the doorknob, creating a minor tear.

Is this the sort of situation that would be stressful to you? Can you think of a time when this scenario would have created a stronger emotional reaction than it does at this moment?

Mood instability is a fact of life for many individuals living with mental health concerns. In a study conducted between April 2006 and March 2013 by South London and Maudsley NHS Trust (SLaM), of 27,704 patients between the ages of 16 and 65, researchers specifically studied the correlation between measurable mood instability and mental disorders. In conclusion, the results found:

Mood instability was documented in 12.1% of people presenting to mental healthcare services. It was most frequently documented in

*people with bipolar disorder (22.6%), but was common in people with
personality disorder (17.8%) and schizophrenia (15.5%).*
- https://www.ncbi.nlm.nih.gov/pmc/articles/PMC4452754/

What Does This Mean for You?

The primary takeaway is that you (or your loved ones) are not alone. If you have found that your moods are cycling faster than you can acknowledge them, or that you often don't realize what type of emotional response you're having until you've had a chance to calm down, you are experiencing something that is common among those who are dealing with mental illness.

Many times, our emotional reactions can also exacerbate our mental health symptoms. People often recall their first panic attack as being absolutely terrifying, not only because the mind and body go into a high alert mode, but because they were unfamiliar with the symptoms they were experiencing. It is not uncommon for people to find out they have GAD in the emergency room, since many of the symptoms that accompany a panic attack– such as shortness of breath and pain in the chest– have been long associated with serious health conditions. The symptoms experienced when your brain steps away from standard operating procedure can be incredibly frightening, ranging from hallucinations, hot/cold flashes, vomiting and diarrhea, panic, erratic behavior, and thoughts of hurting yourself and others. The more terrifying the symptoms, the more emotionally irrational the person experiencing these complaints may become.

Everyone has had a time in their life when they reacted strongly or behaved in a way that later embarrassed them. This might have been in reaction to some important, life-changing news, or a result of too many things happening at once. When you add mental health symptoms to the mix, you can often find your thoughts, emotions, and situations in turmoil and chaos.

Understanding the Emotional/Mental Health Carousel

Does it seem like what you're reading is a bit circular? Do you get the sense that what I've written seems to reiterate what was mentioned at the beginning of this section?

That's the exact type of sensation I'm trying to create here. Mental health and emotional health go hand in hand. One of my mentors once described our emotions as individual horses on a carousel. Some are at the top of their journey, meaning those emotions are very strong, while others cruise along near the floor, meaning they are subdued. However, all the horses continue moving forward in a circular motion, while they crank up and down in patterns that are often hard to decipher. When your mental health is in an ideal state, the carousel horses churn up, down, forward, and back with regularity. When something's wrong with the mechanisms that turn the machine, the horses lurch forward or get frozen in position. The same is true of our emotions when our mental health is suffering.

So, which one comes first? The mental health trigger or the emotional response? And which one are we trying to control? Are we trying to become numbed to triggers or more in control of the emotional response?

The answer is both, though the degree to which we attempt to control triggers or emotional responses can vary from situation to situation, person to person, or even moment to moment.

Like stress, there are some triggers that are helpful to our survival. Being highly averse to touching a stovetop, for example, is beneficial since touching a sizzling hot burner can be extraordinarily painful. If you've ever waved your hand near a burner by accident, the idea of what could happen creates a fear reaction. Those who have been burnt will generally have a stronger response, because their brains equate the stimulus of a burner with the pain and surge of adrenaline that came with that unpleasant experience.

But what if your response to seeing a stovetop is to melt into hysterics, preventing you from even entering a room in which you can see the burners, even if they're not currently hot? Is that weird?

Many people will try to tell you that yes, having that strong of a reaction is weird, and that you need to "get over it." You may have heard that you need to "pull it together," "stop acting spoiled," "don't be a wimp," or "stop making everything about you."

As a response, you'll experience even further negative emotions surrounding the burner stimulus. In addition to giving you a deeply rooted fear and panic, you'll now feel guilty about having such a serious reaction to something other people have no reaction to. You may be embarrassed, and even fall into a self-loathing spiral as you start to focus on more ways in which you perceive yourself to be a failure.

I beg of you, when you reach this place, stop. Stop the freefall. Stop thinking. Slam on the brakes of your emotional descent and allow yourself to look around you.

The stressor, stimulus, or trigger is not always a stovetop burner. That was just a common example that many of us have encountered at some point in our lives. Your trigger could be a certain phrase, situation, color, smell, song, or some type of animal... honestly, anything can be a trigger, depending on the trauma your mind associates with it.

Your trauma is real. Therefore, your emotional response is real. You are feeling the things you are feeling truly and honestly. Every chemical impulse in your body is screaming that these things are a huge problem for your imminent survival, and you need to acknowledge that.

Failure to recognize your emotions just allow you to dig deeper and deeper into the self-hate spiral. "If I weren't crazy, I could do things like other people." "If I weren't such a wimp, I could be successful/have friends/get a partner." All these hateful phrases eventually turn into hateful self-truths, when in fact, they couldn't be further from the truth.

Mental illness is a difficult barrier to maneuver. Like a bad houseguest, it comes out of nowhere, does whatever it wants, eats your leftovers, uses the last of the toilet paper, and steals the batteries to your television remote right before it leaves. It defies logic or control, even in the form of the many helpful medications and therapy options available today.

You can become less sensitive to triggers as time goes by. Working with a professional team of mental health care providers can help you learn to "deal with it," as your well-intending but way out of line friends and family members may put it. But your triggers and your emotions are all real. What we can do is work on how we respond to those emotions and how we react to the situation at the time.

This takes us to our first exercise in which we work to understand what is really happening when we're feeling overwhelmed by our emotions.

Exercise: Untangling Our Emotions

One of the least enjoyable parts of becoming emotional, for many people, is the suddenness with which we can be overtaken by emotion. You're just casually doing whatever you normally do, when out of nowhere a song, memory, or any sort of sensory stimuli comes raging out of nowhere to completely ruin your day.

And then you're left there, violently reacting– or attempting not to react– at the abrupt change in tone from the day. To outside observers, it may look like you've simply "lost it" or are having some type of "conniption fit," as my grandmother attempted to calmly refer to my panic attacks. To them, nothing has happened, but for you, in the heat of the moment, it may actually feel like the world is ending.

Much of our reaction to triggers is involuntary. Our bodies tend to do a lot of things without our express permission, and many of these things are very beneficial. Digestion and breathing are two involuntary processes that we often take for granted because they just happen. But, as anyone who has ever had an upset stomach or practiced yoga can tell you, these involuntary processes are willing to accept a little input from our conscious selves. We can practice diets that help our bodies regulate the chemicals that aid in digestion, and we can learn different breathing techniques to help us get the more air when it's needed the most (there's more detail on that later, I assure you).

The first step to being able to control our reactions is to understand them. And in order to understand our emotions, we must know what we're feeling and when. Unfortunately, when we're in the throes of an emotional reaction, our bodies and brains go on autopilot. Adrenaline can flood the nervous system, forcing all logic and rational thought into the furthest, deepest corners of our brain. You may have heard of the "Four Fs:"

- Fight- in which our bodies respond to stimulus by taking on all threats head on with aggression
- Flight- in which we try to put as much distance between ourselves and the threat
- Freeze- in which we do absolutely nothing
- Fawn- in which we try to charm our way out of perceived danger

Our brain chemicals are responsible for all these reactions, which is really unfortunate since they're not always effective in times of turmoil. However, these were the evolutionary gifts given to us by our ancestors, and we must make do by trying to understand exactly what is happening.

This exercise is not something you can do once and consider yourself cured. If that were the case, I would've been cured in elementary school, because this is an exercise one of my therapists asked me to do all the time.

Instead, this is the type of exercise that you may need to visit frequently, especially when you find yourself having emotions that you don't recognize or that you can't sort out. As mentioned repeatedly, we rarely experience one emotion at a time. In this exercise we'll use different colors to help us sort out what we're feeling, almost like a map of where our brains go when traumatized.

Objectives:
1. Discover all the different things you are feeling when emotions are turbulent. By allowing yourself to freely express these emotions in a tangible way, you'll be able to identify how much of each emotion you are feeling concurrently.
2. To recognize and appreciate when and how you feel emotions concurrently, allowing you to express your emotions and reframe triggering situations through logic.

What You'll Need:

- A piece of blank paper (scrap paper is fine)
- Several different colored crayons, pencils, highlighters, pens, markers... your preferred medium is encouraged
- A safe, quiet place where you can process emotions
- Optional: a support person, animal, or item that brings you comfort
- Optional: a folder in which you can put written exercises for later reference

Here's what you'll do in this exercise:

- Write the date and time somewhere on the piece of paper, along with a brief description of what inspired your current emotional state
- Represent each emotion that you feel with a different colored writing utensil
- Choose whichever color you want for each emotion— you may wish to create a key, so you remember which color is which feeling, but you do not have to
- Use that color to draw out each emotion on the blank piece of paper
- Draw a great big shape to represent emotions that you are feeling strongly
- Color in your shape darker for emotions that are taking control
- Color in lightly the smaller emotions that are tangential to these main emotions

As you work on this exercise, you may find yourself trying to be neat and tidy with your shapes. However, you are not making art. This is not an exercise in perfection. Instead, you are trying to identify your feelings and how they overlap, touch each other, and feed into each other.

It will likely take you a few tries before you feel comfortable doing this exercise completely. In fact, the first few times may feel a bit awkward. Many of us are embarrassed to see all our emotions displayed in a visual, real way. If this is true for you, go ahead and add a swatch that represents your embarrassment.

The purpose of this exercise:

- To help you contextualize your emotions
- To draw a greater understanding of how your emotions manifest
- To connect your emotions to contextual events

Pointers:

- Do not attempt to define the feelings yet. Don't try to sort them out or get involved. Just draw what you feel.
- Don't let yourself think too much the first time you try this. You are not trying to force anything.
- You are not being graded on your artistic talents. A scribble, circle, zig-zag, or any shape is fine, as long as you are being honest with how big and strong it feels.
- It's a good idea to do this exercise when you are feeling a lot of emotions at once. It might not be practical to do it at the height of a triggering episode at first but do it when you can.
- Breathe. Take your time. Allow yourself to sit with your emotions and explore.
- If it becomes too overwhelming at any time, it is completely okay to stop this exercise and seek a form of comfort or support.
- There is no "perfect outcome." Just let your feelings flow through the writing utensil onto the paper.

Release all expectations and get to work. There's really no time limit for this exercise, but once you've been at it for two minutes, stop and look at what you've done. If you feel like adding to your map of emotions, go for it. There is no right or wrong when it comes to scribbling out your feelings on a piece of paper.

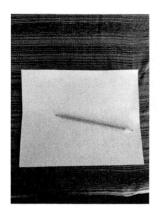 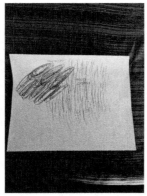 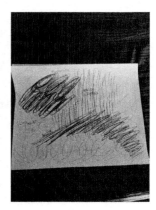

Once you feel satisfied that you've explored your internal emotional landscape as much as you can today, it's time to face your emotions. But first, it's very important to make sure you feel safe doing so.

For many, consciously acknowledging the complexity of our emotions can be difficult. It can be a trigger of its own, especially if you've gotten a lot of criticism for your emotions or how you express them. If you have a member of your support team nearby, you may wish to talk through the results of this exercise with that person.

So, what should you do if you've drawn out all your emotions and don't feel safe?

- Bring out the folder I mentioned earlier when we were gathering supplies for this exercise
- Open the folder and without thinking too much about it, slide in your drawing
- Put the folder in a drawer, bin, closet, or wherever you'll remember it, but not be tempted to force yourself to look at it
- Revisit it when you are ready

Remember that even starting this exercise is a mentally demanding task, and encourage yourself to look at this potential trigger when you're ready. Wanting to face your emotions takes a lot of courage, so putting yourself "out there" so boldly can feel uncomfortable.

When you are ready to look at the visual manifestation of your emotional landscape, try to do so without judging anything. Just look at how big some of the circles are and how small others are. Does anything you see surprise you? What seems familiar?

Now, look at the picture holistically. Can you start to see how the feelings changed as you continued processing the situation? Did some emotions grow while others got smaller? Does it look like you were focused on your emotional response (e.g.- all rage, all joy), or did you find yourself going back to add more and more scribbles as you dug deeper into your emotions?

Again, don't judge yourself for what you see on the paper. You have already felt the emotions. They are already part of reality. You can't go back and "unfeel" them, nor should you. If you were honest with yourself as you drew, you are staring at a pure, deconstructed view of your true emotional reaction to a stimulus. There's nothing shameful about that. Furthermore, no one has to know what you've done or what it means. Does the big yellow circle mean you were feeling jealousy, or is it a representation of the sun? No one but you will know.

You can save these drawings in your folder and compare them to future efforts, or you can destroy them immediately. If I'm trying to work through a particular issue, I tend to keep them so that I can assure myself that emotions can change, and feelings can heal and grow. For example, I had a breakup that churned out a rather stunning portfolio of hurt and anger.

On the other hand, if I'm doing it just because I need to sort out what I'm feeling now, I generally get rid of them. I remember one incident when I was deeply triggered by a basket full of clean, unfolded laundry due to childhood trauma. I completely shut down, which frightened me, because this trigger hadn't manifested in decades.

Out came the paper and crayons, and I drew a brilliant landscape of circles that represented anger, self-loathing, regret, shame, guilt, sadness, and jealousy. Looking at it, I discovered that my reaction to being triggered was stronger than the actual triggering situation. That is, I was experiencing strong emotions about my trauma, but I was more upset that I was having strong emotions!

One of the reasons I enjoy this exercise is because it can help you organize all those complexities. Like the characters in the Harry Potter example, we sometimes don't understand all the feelings we're having until we finally hit the point at which we can no longer be stoic. Once I realized that I was mostly upset about my perceived "weakness" for being triggered, I was able to focus on accepting the triggering situation. As a result, I could validate my emotions, understand why I was triggered, and re-approach the basket of laundry without being blindsided by my emotions.

Reminders:

- You will not be "cured" doing this once.
- If you feel that you have done it wrong, you have not.
- We view different scenarios through different lenses depending on our mood/mind frame. If you revisit your drawings, do not judge your past self for having these emotions. They were real at the time, and now you've moved on.

Once you have completed this activity, here are a few questions you can ask yourself:

- What does this tell me about how I responded to this emotional state?
- How do these emotions impact my train of thought as I process an event/trigger/stimulus?
- How did these emotions inspire how I reacted physically to the event/trigger/stimulus?
- What parts of this experience did I not enjoy?
- Are there areas in which I could potentially coax my emotions into relaxing a bit, so I can process the event/trigger/stimulus without reacting in a way that I do not wish to react?

Don't allow yourself to become stuck on the idea of "I shouldn't have acted this way" or "I shouldn't have felt this way." Your actions, reactions, and emotions are all valid at the time they are experienced. We do this exercise so we can recognize patterns and learn to reframe our responses, not shame ourselves about how our minds and bodies automatically react to things that are outside of our control.

If this exercise is not ideal for you right now, make note of it, and refer to it in another setting, when you might be feeling confused or overwhelmed by your emotional response to a situation. It's always waiting for you.

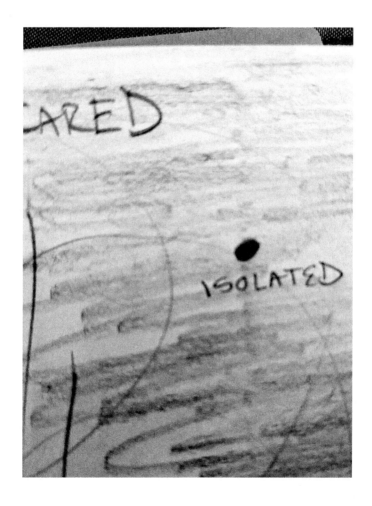

GETTING ON TRACK FOR TAKING CONTROL OF YOUR EMOTIONAL HEALTH

Now that we've had the opportunity to meditate on how our emotions resonate within us during times when our mental health is not at its best, let's move forward to look at how our mental health is right now.

Because of the nature of this book, you may be reading this section on a good day, a bad day, or even on a pretty decent, neutral day. So, before we get started on our next set of activities, let me ask again:

How do you feel? How have you felt today? How are you feeling right now?

Most of the time, we take our mood for granted, especially if we're in a neutral space. These are the types of days where you might not feel like you're in the best of spirits, but you're certainly not feeling terrible. Your activity level could range from busy to bored, but the key common denominator of these days is that you are emotionally neutral. Nothing to see here— just being yourself and doing your thing.

On the other hand, there are days where you're definitely feeling something. This may be in response to a trigger or stimulus, as we discussed in the last section, or it may be because your brain has decided today is the day to "Feel All The Things."

What I mean by "Feel All The Things" is just that– your mind decides to throw all your emotions in a bag, shake it up, and dump it on the floor. Usually there's not a reason for this event. That's the beauty of mental illness. Whether you live with the high-tensile thrum of anxiety or the dripping despair of depression, there are days when your emotions seem like too much to handle.

When we have those days, we can often trace them back to the source and dissect them with the exercise we completed in the last chapter. But sometimes, we aren't in a good head space to really drill down into the nitty gritty of why and how we're feeling the emotions we are.

On those days, we need to instead take a moment to look at our overall current mental health status. How often do you have those "Feel All The Things" days? Do you have them more frequently than not? Or would you say instead that most of your days go by without serious incident, but every once in a while– boy oh boy– it just really hits you all at once?

One way we can get in touch with any patterns in our emotional state is to learn how to inspect our current mental health status. Taking stock of how we're feeling regularly can help us in many ways– let's check it out together.

Looking at Your Current Mental Health Status

Because of the waxing, waning, and sometimes unpredictable nature of our mental health status, many experts recommend keeping a journal so that you can keep up with all the changes or lack of changes in your mental and emotional health.

However, we're also aware that mental and emotional health are not a "one-thing-helps-all" sort of situation. Journaling can be a very therapeutic mindfulness activity for some, but a very stressful forced activity for others. As a result, some people have an even greater adverse emotional reaction to this task than others.

As someone with mental health issues, you've probably heard people tell you to "just get over it" or "do it anyway" when it comes to completing a task that causes you significant emotional strife. Sometimes this can be helpful advice, especially when your physical safety is at risk.

Example:
Joe would really like to cross a busy street, but to do so, he'll need to tap the pedestrian signal button in the crosswalk. Joe under-stands that many people have touched the button before him, and the idea of touching it is very uncomfortable to him.

Unfortunately, this is a situation in which Joe must do something he is uncomfortable with in order to complete a specific activity. This is the type of situation where telling someone to "do it anyway" might be appropriate, though we can come up with some more encouraging ways to go about it!

The goal of any exercise that connects your consciousness to your emotional and mental status is not to bombard you with negative feelings. Instead, it's intended to help you understand and track your mental health status. Of course, any event in which you really dig into your mental health has the potential to set things off, so let's start casually.

Here are a few questions you can ask yourself:
- How is it going right now?
- What is going well right now?
- Where do I need some help right now?

There may be times when you feel unprepared to answer these questions, and that's ok. Maybe when you ask yourself these questions, you don't have an answer right away– and that's also okay. However, try to get in the habit of checking in with yourself at strategic times throughout the day such as first thing in the morning or when you're noticing a shift in your mood.

From here, you can build the conversation a bit more. Perhaps instead of looking at how things are going at this exact moment, you can look at the entire day. How was your day? What went well today? What were some challenging moments that occurred today? Add on to this last question with "and how did I get through it?"

This can be challenging, because many of us don't want to relive our day, especially if it was exceptionally difficult. We've become accustomed to answering the question "How are you?" or "How was your day?" with "Fine, thanks. And you?" That's because many of us associate this type of inquiry as a formality, not an actual desire to know how things are going. But when you're the one asking yourself these questions, it's okay to be completely honest.

Sometimes, we consider doing things like journaling to be stressful because we must face our emotions and challenges. The truth is, we always have to face our emotions and challenges, but if it doesn't feel right to put those things on paper, you don't have to. While keeping track of these feelings is important, if you don't feel safe writing things out where you or other people might find them, don't. There are other options.

Therefore, let's try doing this in a less concrete, not-so-confrontational way. You can start by asking yourself how it's going several times a day. Then, when you're comfortable, check in with yourself at the end of the day.

Don't dwell on how you could've done better. Absolutely anyone can look at their day with the perfect vision of hindsight and explain a thousand things they wish they'd done differently. That's simply the nature of living. "The only people who get to plot all of their actions and verbal responses perfectly are fictional characters," a therapist once explained to me, and it's very true. What we say and do throughout the day is spontaneous, built on our physical, mental, intellectual, and emotional capacity at the time, so try to avoid a step-by-step replay of your day, and focus instead on how you felt. Were you confident? Sleepy? Stressed? Okay? Was there a time when your emotional state changed? Why was that? How did you feel as you worked through that?

Then, you can start to look at your wellbeing in chunks of time. Notice when you've had a few consecutive days of relatively good mental health. Or make it a point to notice when you've been in a streak of particularly foul moods. You may choose to mark these periods on a calendar to help you see if there are any notable patterns.

Example:

Wendy's coworkers are always joking about how it must be "that time of the month" because she's very emotional at the beginning of each month. This makes Wendy angry, because her heightened emotions have nothing to do with menstruation, and she doesn't understand why her coworkers are mocking her when she's clearly having a difficult time.

She starts to track the days when she experiences the most emotional outbursts and realizes that they occur at the end of the month and during the first week of the month. Looking at some of the stressful things in her life, she realizes this is when all her bills are due. Is it possible that some of Wendy's emotional challenges are related to the stress she feels over her financial situation?

Important dates or anniversaries, deadlines, changes in the weather, physical stressors, and hormonal cycles can all have an impact on our mental health and emotional state. While not every triggering situation will have a clear and direct cause, it's not a bad idea to keep track of these dates and your emotional state leading up to and following them. This can help give you insight into how you may be responding to these triggers— or failing to ignore them.

Checking in with yourself every so often is a great way to reconnect with how you're feeling. In our fast-paced culture, we're often encouraged to ignore our emotions and mental health triggers so that we can get things done. As a result, many of us pack our feelings away so we can acknowledge them at a more convenient time.

Unfortunately, there's rarely a good time to process emotions that aren't so enjoyable. Much like any other task we ignore for too long, failing to empty the emotional storage bin can be just as problematic as dealing with an overflowing garbage can – things can get messy.

Therefore, a daily or even weekly check in can be a good routine to help you discover those less enjoyable emotions before the bin tips over and spills everywhere.

This is also a good time to ask yourself what you're doing to help your mental and emotional state and uncover what coping skills might not be so helpful.

What Is Working?

When you ask yourself "what is working," you're trying to identify key things that you have consciously or subconsciously done to help boost your mental and emotional health. This can include things like:

- Going for a walk instead of engaging in a fight
- Doing yoga when you start to get frustrated
- Allowing yourself to cry when you get overwhelmed
- Deep, intentional breathing when your mind starts to race

These are all significant choices we can make to divert our emotional energy when our mental health isn't at its best. But some of the things we do every day help us engage in a more positive emotional state, too. Consider things like:

- Making a cup of your favorite beverage just the way you like it in the morning
- Putting up a picture you enjoy at your desk
- Taking the time to listen to a song you really like on the way to work
- Paying someone a compliment

It may seem that these insignificant activities have nothing to do with your emotional health, but really, they're all ways that you sub-consciously work to make yourself happy. Taking the time to add a little honey to your morning tea might seem like an automatic action, but you're doing it because you want to. You are taking an elective step towards making yourself happy, and that's a good thing.

Ask yourself:

- What is the best part of my day?
- What do I do when I'm feeling stressed?
- What are some behaviors I really enjoy?
- How do I reward myself when things go well?
- Do I reward myself often enough?
- What are my most healthful behaviors and how do they make me feel?

These are just a few questions that can help you discover what is currently helping your overall mental health status. Don't dwell on whether your answers are "good enough" or even good at all. This is just a way to identify what you're doing right now to keep negative emotions and bad mental health days at bay.

Example:

Years ago, I worked at an insurance agency. One day I noticed that my coworker and I would have a hearty snack of cheese and crackers around 3pm every day. We would bring in multiple types of cheese and crispy treats to share. Eventually the entire office started joining us for snack hour.

When we stopped to really think about it, we realized that this was our way of rewarding ourselves for getting through the most stressful part of the day. After 3pm, the walk-in traffic subsided, and we could get our administrative work done with minimal interruptions. Our "Cheese Breaks" gave us something to look forward to after hours of absorbing the wrath of angry, frustrated customers.

Gorging ourselves on cheese probably wasn't the most healthful way to explore our emotions or boost our mental health, but it was clear that we needed some type of event in our day to help us maintain our composure.

What types of things do you do to help you focus on keeping your mental health in tip-top shape? How do these activities or behaviors change when you're having a bad day?

Sometimes we don't recognize the things we do to help ourselves cope with regular stresses. Now is a good time to check in and think about everything that you are doing in your life to increase your mood and improve your emotional state.

Mini-Activity: What Works?

What You'll Need: A piece of paper and a writing utensil.

What You'll Do: Make a list of all the things you do to help yourself, mentally and emotionally.

Objective: To understand what coping mechanisms you are currently using to help you with mental and emotional health issues.

Take the time to consider everything you do regularly that you enjoy or have committed to as part of your wellness routine.

When you feel confident that the list you have made is a thorough, picture of all the happy spots in your day or week and look at what you've written down.

Reminder: This could include regular daily activities, like eating cheese or starting the day with some exercise. It could also take the form of treating yourself to a favorite lunch or special coffee drink when the day has been particularly rough. Sometimes the positive things we do to help ourselves cope can be as simple as taking a few mindful deep breaths or splashing some water on our face to help us stay in the moment.

Take a few moments to review the list. What are your thoughts? How do you feel about this list?

One interesting thing that many people– including myself– find when completing this exercise is how many little things we do to help ourselves feel "okay." Maybe you have a favorite blanket or a television show you like to watch when your emotions are particularly volatile. Some therapists have observed patients returning to a familiar book or movie when they're not sure how stable they are feeling emotionally– without consciously realizing that they are seeking the comfort that comes from immersing yourself in something you know.

We tend to seek out rewards and consolation to help us stay on a stable emotional path. These may be edible, drinkable, musical, recreational, spiritual, or physical. If you enjoy it, chances are you have found a way to incorporate this pleasure into your regular routine, either to fortify your strength in getting through a day that has been tough emotionally and mentally, or to cocoon yourself in happy feelings when things have gone terribly.

The next step is to evaluate how each of these activities, techniques, or rituals benefits us when we're in a highly emotional state. This is not a matter of judging yourself on the choices you make but gauging whether each behavior is effectively changing your mental or emotional health status. Using my example above, one could argue that a cheese buffet has terrible health ramifications and could be replaced by a more healthful behavior. However, the focus of this exercise is to see what works, and I would unequivocally say that our office cheese parties helped keep us all sane and functioning through long, stressful days.

Therefore, don't let yourself consider whether you should be doing these things, but whether they help you.

Note: If you are not able to walk away from any feelings of shame or doubt you have about your list, then I recommend putting the list away or destroying it and talking to your mental health professional about what you found worrisome. As I mentioned in the early pages of this book, sometimes exploration of our emotions can uncover some gnarly issues. Once again, if you feel uncomfortable or emotionally worse when doing these exercises, immediately stop and connect with your care team. We're not here to start a crisis; we're here to understand ourselves mentally and emotionally so we can move forward and reframe our emotional responses into neutral- and eventually positive- experiences.

Now that you know what exercises, activities, and behaviors are helpful, what should you do with that information? The short answer is "Do more of it!"

This is, of course, within reason. You do not need to perform 24 consecutive hours of yoga in order to feel the benefits it can have for your mind and body. Instead, consider taking short breaks throughout the day to stretch and move meaningfully. This could mean doing a chair pose next to your desk chair or doing a few stretches while practicing mindful breathing during a break.

Similarly, if your special coffee drink is your bliss, consuming it relentlessly will not elevate your mood or improve your emotional status. Quite the opposite is generally true when it comes to an overload of caffeine and sugar. Instead, appreciate the routine for how it makes you feel. Order your personalized drink with a smile, knowing that you are taking time to appreciate yourself, and that you are enjoying this coffee because you enjoy taking care of yourself.

Putting a mindful spin on some of your regular activities can really deepen your connection to the restorative nature of the activity. The knowledge that you are really trying to take care of yourself in times of strife can be more powerful than the stress that is causing your emotional state. While the triggers may be strong and the trauma seems unbearable, you are moving forward with trying to create a safe and enjoyable space for yourself. That dedication to your well-being deserves celebration!

There may be scenarios in which "more" might mean "higher quality," rather than "more frequently."

Example:
Going to the gym to vent your feelings on the emotionless exercise equipment is a great way to treat your mind to some release. However, if you're working out to the point where your body crosses the threshold between "hurts so good" and "hurts so bad," you might be approaching your strategy from a negative point of view. Furthermore, going to the gym every time you're in a difficult emotional headspace may lead to constantly working out, which then starts pushing into realms of addiction. Don't compound your problem and

focus on quality before quantity.

Instead of using exercise to "punish" yourself for feeling things you didn't want to feel, or for lashing out, or other harsh responses to a challenging situation, concentrate on what you enjoy about exercise. Some people enjoy the rush of endorphins, or consider the time spent at the gym or studio as "me time" to reflect upon and analyze their thoughts.

It's not a bad idea to ask yourself "what about this do I like?" especially if it's not immediately obvious. You might shock yourself by discovering that you don't have an emotional connection to an item on your list. That's okay– right now we're focusing on things that *are* working for you, so hold onto that so we can unpack what's *not* working next.

Consider how each activity benefits you, and ways you can increase your participation with it. Approach this from the standpoint of making each day better so that you can establish a mindful habit to practice when things get rough.

Please note that I'm not suggesting that taking a few deep breaths, drinking coffee, or going to the gym is going to bring any mental or emotional breakdown to a screeching halt. This will not remove or eliminate any of your emotions.

Instead, the goal of this exercise is to help you recognize the things that bring you pleasure when you are in the most pain, then mindfully approach these things when your emotions run high. When you feel triggered, or more emotional than you were prepared to be at that moment, think of your list of "Things That Work" to help you feel positive.

You may come up empty handed when trying to find something simple to quell the storm inside your mind, but you'll have bought yourself thirty seconds to step inside your own mind rather than experiencing a sudden outburst.

Example:

One of my favorite soothing treats is green tea with honey in it. While my English grandparents would be dismayed to know I said this, tea can't entirely solve every problem. However, when I feel like something is amiss with my mental or emotional state, I ask myself if I need to make a cup of tea.

Most of the time, the cup of tea never gets made. Instead, I look inside to see what's not right. Am I feeling anxious, overwhelmed, or angry at what my emotions are dictating? What needs attention right now?

It has taken me ten years to train myself to understand this cue reasonably well, so don't expect to wake up with a new perspective on life. However, knowing that something works helps me remember that I won't be feeling these emotions forever, and that I really need to stop and sort things out before my mental health takes a significant dive.

Striking a balance between emotion and logic is not easy. There will still be times when holding your tears, temper, or laughter will be impossible. However, practicing these exercises can help you appreciate when and how you can use the things you enjoy in your life to hold you in reality, even when your emotions want to run wild.

What's Not Working?

Once you've sorted out a few things that are working to boost and amplify your mental health and emotional wellness, it's time to reflect on the things that aren't helping you on your journey to elevate your overall well-being.

This part can be especially painful because of the many dimensions "not helpful" can take. As with my cheese example, it could be that your reward or encouraging behavior isn't exactly healthful. Over-indulging in anything can become harmful, especially if you are participating in this behavior to avoid or punish yourself for your negative thoughts and emotions, as pointed out with the gym example.

However, at the beginning of your emotional and mental health self-discovery voyage, you may find yourself in an "all or nothing" mentality. This is often the first step for those battling addictive behaviors, or those trying to eliminate something that has become problematic in other ways.

Example:
Lee has been stopping at the farmer's market on the way home from work. Lee buys a bouquet of fresh-cut flowers which they take home and arrange neatly in a vase. The next morning, Lee throws away the previous night's bouquet to make way for the new one they'll purchase tonight.

This behavior is not harmful and brings Lee great joy. However, they have noticed that the bouquets are becoming increasingly expensive, and they're finding more and more faults in the flowers. The act of picking out a bouquet has now become stressful to Lee, yet they feel that if they stop doing it, something bad is going to happen.

In this scenario, the behavior of purchasing a new bouquet could be seen as not resourceful, or even wasteful but not necessarily harmful, as the bouquets would exist regardless of Lee's presence. However, the fact that buying flowers has become stressful for Lee indicates that it is no longer serving a purpose for them.

This might be a case where it's time to put an end to the behavior. Sure, it's not as bad as some addictions, but Lee is starting to have negative feelings towards their own behavior. That's a sign that it's not working.

There are many other signs that one or more of your current coping mechanisms may not be working as well as you think it is. These signs can include:

- You are spending more time and energy on your coping behavior than other areas of your life
- The amount of money you are spending is overwhelming your household budget
- You are avoiding other situations in your life so you can enjoy your coping behavior
- You are avoiding certain people in your life because you know they would not approve

- You feel personal shame about what you're doing and try to "hide" it
- You are starting to seek increasingly difficult, expensive, opulent, or dangerous ways of performing this behavior
- You have noticed a significant change in your health that can be directly attributed to this action
- You no longer enjoy the activity, but you feel like you are being forced to do it as part of your routine

While these attributes are often associated with serious situations such as drug, alcohol, gambling, or sex addiction, it is possible to experience these negative sensations with any behavior or activity. These are all signs that it is a good time to move away from this activity for the time being.

Mini Activity: It's Just Not Working Anymore!

Let's take a look at the list you made during the last mini activity. We originally examined this list through the lens of what was going well– what is actually working for you and keeping you mentally healthy and your emotions in check.

Now let's look at it with a slightly less positive gaze. What are some things you'd like to cross off the list? This doesn't mean excluding activities that are "bad" for you but rather things that simply aren't working anymore.

As in Lee's example, your coping activities may not be detrimental to your health or mental, emotional, financial, or personal wellness, but they just may not be bringing you pleasure anymore. In instances such as these, it's not a bad idea to really examine what you're doing and why.

Example:

After several months of increasingly opulent cheese buffets, my coworkers and I realized that we were taking this a bit overboard. Every day was becoming a gourmet-level potluck. We were skipping lunch and moving our cheese feast to earlier in the day as a result. Soon, the cheese had nothing to do with boosting our morale throughout the workday and became a way for us to bond over every cranky customer.

While our team was never closer than when we were venting about difficult customers around plates of cheese, we were all feeling the effects. Our clothes were fitting a little tighter. Our paychecks were going towards snacks instead of healthy meals. Furthermore, we no longer felt relief when we brought out the cheese– just an overwhelming dread as to how terrible the day was going to be after a particularly difficult customer.

It was clear that we needed to reassess the situation.

I know that we just discussed "do more of what works"; one of the dangers of doing what works more is that we become reliant on that behavior or activity to make us feel better all the time.

Sometimes, this isn't a bad thing. If playing with your household pet is helpful for maintaining control over your emotional state and helping you find a good baseline in your mental health, then you have a nice activity to look forward to. However, if you find yourself experiencing negative emotions when your pet decides not to play with you, or you're skipping work or school to spend time with your pet, that's a good indicator that your "do more" has transcended into "not working" territory.

Most of the activities on your list will not be this cut and dry. You may find some things on your list that you do, but don't find helpful.

Example:

Journaling is one of the most highly recommended activities for individuals with mental illnesses and emotional difficulties. Writing your thoughts and emotions in a journal can be a great way to connect with the reality of what you are feeling versus what you are actually experiencing and can offer everyone a safe platform on which they can really work out their often complicated thoughts.

However, there are many people– myself included– who feel very anxious about journaling. Perhaps you have had your privacy invaded in the past, or you are fearful about going back and reading what you've written because you know you'll try to shame yourself for irrational behavior.

For many years, I tried to journal because that's what my therapists recommended. Thankfully, we live in an age where more interventions are readily available, so when I shared with my most recent therapist that I barely tolerate journaling, she recommended I stop immediately.

When we are forced to do things that do not serve us, we often experience an entirely new crop of negative emotions related to that task. Sometimes we need a little extra push to help us through a particularly stubborn moment. However, modern mental health experts are now recognizing that sometimes if we don't want to do a particular task, there is an actual emotional or mental health-related factor involved. Perhaps the activity you're being asked to do relates back to triggers or trauma from earlier in your life. It is also possible that the feelings of guilt or displeasure you have at doing a certain activity can overwhelm you mentally or emotionally.

Therefore, when you consider the items on your list that are not working, don't simply exclude things that might be considered "bad habits" or "overkill." Instead, truly consider each item to determine whether it is serving you properly.

Ask yourself additional questions such as:
Do I really enjoy this, or do I feel obligated to do it?
When I complete this activity, do I feel more balanced, optimistic, or calm?
What part of this activity helps me the most?
What changes in my mental and emotional status when I work on this activity?
Would I recommend this to a friend or family member?
Have I discussed this activity with my mental health care team?

Your answers to these questions can help you determine if you need to remove a behavior from your list. Bear in mind that while the concept of "do or do not" can feel very polarizing and harsh, there are ways to incorporate aspects of that activity you have really enjoyed as you continue prioritizing your mental and emotional health. While my daily cheese buffets are a thing of the past, I'm still known to incorporate a tasty nibble of cheese into my particularly rough days. It reminds me that I've overcome a much more difficult barrage of stressful situations, and that I deserve something to enjoy after my emotional and mental battles.

We all deserve a way to take care of ourselves in a way that makes sense to us. Think of your mental health as being like your physical health. For example, while many of us don't particularly love brushing our teeth, it makes sense that we need to scrub the plaque and debris from our teeth each day in order to keep our mouths healthy. As a result, we typically do what we can to make our oral healthcare routine more enjoyable– we choose toothpastes and mouthwashes that we enjoy, toothbrushes that are comfortable in our mouths, and so on. Many people sing a little song in their head or set timers to make sure they're brushing their teeth the correct amount of time. It's all the process of making something necessary less stressful.

Therefore, when you think about the activities that keep you mentally and emotionally healthy, keep yourself in the mindset of making it as enjoyable as possible. Just as you would stop using a toothpaste that you found intolerable, it may be time to end your relationship with activities that are not helping you facilitate the level of mental and emotional health you desire.

So, why can't you just end your relationship with whatever is stressing you out? If your job is so stressful that you're eating a ton of cheese, why don't you just leave the job?

For many of us, these decisions aren't simple. Very few of us can walk away from our main source of income without preparing for a shift in financial status. If you find specific people or situations triggering, you may wish to avoid them. However, this can be extremely difficult and cause even greater stress as you feel trapped or inconvenienced by your own mental health.

Part of functioning in a fast-paced, stressful world as people with mental illness and emotional health considerations is knowing what works and what doesn't work when it comes to coping with your triggers and traumas. It's never a bad idea to have your emotional coping toolbox full of potential tools that you can use when an unexpected event occurs. Unfortunately, we don't know what works until we try it, which is why it's important to go through your toolbox and consider what is currently working and not working, just as we have in these two mini-activities.

Often, we find that we fall back on familiar habits. We do what we know best because it has worked in the past. Funny little habits like picking at your fingernails and fidgeting with a particular object or a sensory tool are deep-seated coping mechanisms that we may per-form without even noticing. Most of the time, these have no negative impact on the way we function, but when they do become a problem, they can have a negative effect on how we continue to grow and maintain our emotional and mental health.

Therefore, it's not a bad idea to take a few moments to complete these mini exercises once in a while to ensure you're cognizant of not only what is and isn't working, but why. Upon further contemplation, you might discover that change is necessary.

Brainstorm: Discovering New Territory

If reframing our emotions, changing our mind, and eliminating undesired behaviors was easy, we'd live in a very different world. Imagine if one day, a life-long smoker could throw away their last pack of cigarettes, say, "well, I guess I'm done with that," and live the rest of their lives as though they'd never been addicted to nicotine. Likewise, imagine if you could say, "I guess I'm done getting angry!" and never have to worry about the ramifications of that emotion ever again.

Regardless of the behavior we're attempting to modify, it's going to be difficult. You might find yourself experiencing a brand-new range of difficult and negative emotions. This may cause you to long for "the old way." Your mind and body may also argue with you, insisting that the status quo was actually just fine, and we really don't need to put all this effort into the new way.

Change is very disruptive to many people, regardless of any emotional or mental illness challenges they may experience.

> *Example:*
> *Fran is a top-level executive who hardly misses a minute of work, much less a whole day. After undergoing a minor medical procedure, she returns to the office the next day feeling very anxious. In her first few meetings of the day, she has to*

be reminded of various targets and project scopes. She feels completely discombobulated and even shows up late to a few weekly meetings later in the day.

Fran may feel like she's losing her mind, but she's experiencing a pretty normal reaction to change.

Whether or not they actively enjoy their routines, most people appreciate the regularity of performing certain tasks at certain times and knowing exactly what is expected of them at all moments. In a world where it seems like everything that matters is beyond our control, a routine can help us feel empowered. We know what's going on, what's going to happen, and what we can do to temporarily modify that situation in any way.

Any time we experience a significant change in our routine, our brains and bodies tend to scream, "Hey! Wait! This isn't right!" We may experience any of the Four Fs mentioned earlier. We might forget automatic patterns– such as showing up for a weekly meeting– or finer details that we typically have committed to memory– like the scope of a current project.

Therefore, when folks say, "change is hard," it goes beyond being in a bad mood because you can't have something you want. Willpower and determination are part of the equation, but you can only change what you want to change.

We'll look more at what it takes to change our emotional behavior in the next chapter, but while we're examining our current coping activities, it might be a good time to brainstorm the type of future we want to have. Ultimately, our main goal is to be more in tune to our emotions and mental health status as well as our potential response to situations that challenge our wellness. But in order to get there, we need to put more tools in our toolbox, especially if we just took a few out in the last mini activity.

This is a good time to consider what behaviors might help you cope with emotionally charged situations that challenge your mental health.

Objectives:
- To explore new behaviors that might help you mitigate situations during which your mental and emotional health might be challenged
- To carefully consider things that you enjoy or feel can assist you on your journey

What You'll Need:
- A system for keeping notes, e.g. notebook, spreadsheet, dry erase board. .
- Access to the internet or a library. There will be research involved.
- A support person to bounce ideas back and forth with you.

What You'll Do in This Exercise:
- Think of all the things you would like to try. Everything is a valid option from something grand like skydiving to something small like learning how to write your name on a grain of rice.
- Don't think of whether they're practical, and don't worry about how you'll do them. That's the next step, so for now, focus on what you would like to try.

- Jot down all the things you think of that you might like to investigate further.

Based on what you have discovered does and does not work to help you connect to and appreciate your emotional and mental state during volatile times, you are looking for new tools to add to your toolbox.

Brainstorm a few activities that you think you might like to pursue. This could include hobbies, crafts, exercises, or activities. They may be brand new to you or a different spin on a familiar behavior. For example, those who enjoy playing fetch with their dog might consider taking their dog on a walk regularly. This is still considered a "new" behavior, even if interacting with the dog might be very familiar.

The Purpose of This Exercise:
- To help you brainstorm activities that can help you rediscover balance when you are at your most emotional
- To add more tools to your mental health and emotional support tool box
- To find behaviors that are healthful and helpful

Pointers:
- Don't spend too much time deliberating whether you should or shouldn't add something to your list of prospective activities. This is not a binding contract– just a brainstorm!
- Don't feel the need to write a comprehensive list in just one attempt. You can continue your brainstorm over several days or weeks.

Try to think of a range of activities, from things you can do anytime and anywhere, to things you can look forward to enjoying once your emotional state has passed. Additionally, consider different types of exercises:

- Sensory activities allow you to use sight, touch, taste, sound, and smell to help diffuse your emotional state, and are often good "quick fixes" for reframing an anxious and emotional mind.

- Creative activities involve making and changing things. Sometimes, when we feel out of control, producing something tangible– whether a craft or a clean closet– can make us feel a little more connected with our mind, body, and environment.

- Brain and body activities require mental and physical prowess. These can be wonderful ways to redirect our thoughts into a constructive and positive space so we can reconnect with our reality when emotions are high. Remember to respect the fine line that exists between challenging yourself and overwhelming yourself. We all move, learn, and grow at different paces.

- Relaxing activities are just that - creating a space where you can fully relax. Regardless of what our emotional landscape looks like, our bodies often respond to emotion with tension. The physical effects of tension are very real and can be quite painful for many people, so helping your body feel safe to relax can be physically and mentally essential.

Here are just a few examples from each category to help you with your brainstorming process. These are presented in no particular order and were acquired from surveying my mentors and acquaintances who struggle with mental and emotional illness:

Sensory

Cuddling with a pet

Engaging with a fidget tool or toy

Calm Strips

Aromatherapy

Sitting/walking/observing nature

Listening to music

Looking at art

Reading

Looking through old photos

Creating

Crafting

Needlework/Knitting/Crocheting

Baking/Cooking

Painting/Drawing

Gardening

Organizing your home

Improving the home/DIY

Writing

Doing puzzles

Brain and Body

Going for a walk

Yoga

Mindful stretching

Going to the gym

Taking your dog for a walk/playing with your dog

Doing household chores

Volunteering with a local organization

Tutoring

Taking a class to learn a new skill

Traveling

Learning to play a game

Word puzzles

Relaxing

Meditation

Taking a hot bath or shower

Taking a nap

Practicing self-care

Trying Yoga Nidra

Watching a familiar movie or television program

Creating a cocoon, pillow fort, or other safe place to practice mindfulness

Relaxation apps

Reminders:

- There is no wrong way to perform this exercise.
- None of these activities are intended to "fix" you and your issues. They are intended to be focal points that you can consider when you find yourself overwhelmed by triggers and emotions.

Once you have completed this activity, it's time to take it to the next level. Take a look at the list you have created and start researching what it would take to actually be involved in some of these activities. This means looking around your home, considering the amount of time necessary to practice these activities in your daily schedule, finding the right resources, and in some cases, learning a little bit about what each activity entails.

Here are a couple examples of how you can organize your research for each potential activity:

Activity: Doing puzzles
What you will need: Puzzles and a large table
Is it affordable: Yes
How much time do you need to devote to it: As much as desired
Can I do this anywhere: No, not portable
Will there be immediate gratification: Only if the trigger occurs at home

Activity: Learning to play chess
Pros: Requires a lot of thought, can help me focus, not expensive, good for the brain
Cons: Requires a partner, who do I know that can teach me chess? Matches can last a long time, do I really want to concentrate that much? No immediate gratification

Activity: Listening to music
What I like: Can be done anywhere with or without headphones. Can learn more about music and make it a hobby. Can always listen to my favorite music. Good for helping with

mindful breathing and movement. I have a lot of great albums at home I can listen to.

What I don't like: Sometimes I get sensitive to sound when triggered. Sometimes I don't know what I want to listen to and that makes me feel grumpier. There's a lot of music out there, which is kind of overwhelming. I don't know where to start, but I don't want to listen to the same stuff over and over again.

However you choose to organize your thoughts and feelings about the activities you have listed is perfectly fine as long as you are honest with yourself.

One idea is to come up with a few different categories for activities you can start right away, those that will take a little research or extra resources and supplies (such as learning a new skill or crafting), those that may not be practical right now, but you don't want to eliminate, and those that are just not a good idea. Again, this is not a legal contract, so it's okay to change your mind.

Once you've organized your thoughts regarding all the activities you might be able to pursue, it's time to take them seriously. Try them out. Don't just try the activity when you're feeling great, but when you're very stressed as well.

Go at your own pace. Don't try to force yourself into doing something that doesn't feel right. Think of these as tools that you can put in your mental and emotional wellness toolbox. Just as a hammer isn't the correct tool for every task, playing with your dog won't help every high-stress emotional state. Give yourself grace to try and fail, try and kind of succeed, and try again. Furthermore, if it doesn't work, don't feel bad about your decision to try. No one is wonderful at everything, and everyone must practice something many times before they get even close to "doing it right." Mistakes will be made, but knowledge and mindfulness will be gained.

Frequently ask yourself, "is this working?" Once you've managed to put your finger on what is limiting your success, ask yourself why that roadblock is occurring. Check in with yourself frequently to determine whether your coping behavior or activity is really doing anything beneficial for you.

If that last paragraph sounds familiar, that's because this is a very cyclical exercise. Sometimes you find hobbies and activities you love forever. Sometimes they only benefit you for a while. The process of gaining insight into your mental and emotional health involves constant growth into a mindful state. And, just as a child's clothes are left behind while the body grows, some of your mindfulness tools won't be used as much as you continue to make progress. Therefore, it is natural to repeat this whole pattern from, "is this serving me?" to, "what should I be doing?" many times in your life.

You may have to repeat to yourself many times, **"This is not going to fix me but help me navigate my mental and emotional territory when things get rough."** Set reasonable expectations for yourself, and always remember that your emotions are valid and how you express them is natural. However, if you feel that your emotional response is disrupting the life you want to live, putting these tools into your toolbox can help you thrive.

PREPARING FOR CHANGE

As much as we would like to say "ready, set, go" and have all our dreams come true, the world simply doesn't work like that. Some changes are easier to make than others. In fact, incorporating big and little changes into your life can be equally difficult or simple.

Unfortunately, we don't know exactly how hard change is going to be until we start the process. That's why, for many people, preparing for change can be just as important as fully incorporating new patterns and behaviors in your life.

The stages of change include:
1. Precontemplation
2. Contemplation
3. Preparation
4. Action
5. Maintenance
6. Relapse

Chances are high that you were in the precontemplation or contemplation stage when you picked up this book. You may have recognized that your mental and emotional health had been lagging, and even though you weren't quite sure what to do about it, you had a sneaking suspicion that your life would be better if you did something about it. But, like many aspects of our lives, you may have found yourself overwhelmed with some other responsibility and let your mental health fall to the wayside.

The first few chapters of this book have been dedicated to getting you through the contemplation state, in which you start to imagine a new future and give serious consideration to what you are willing to do in order to make changes in your life to benefit your mental and emotional status. Yes, these are intended to be tools to help you manage your behavior and mental health when emotions run high, but change is still change, especially if you are adopting these new tools to replace activities that are no longer helping you.

Have you ever tried to make a change before? Perhaps you've adopted a new diet, tried a budget-friendly household product, or tried to change your schedule. It may seem like "no big deal" on paper, but it can be hard to remember new details, no matter how significant. This alone can be triggering for those who live with mental illnesses. Therefore, before we jump in the water and try new tools, it's a good idea to get prepared for the action.

What Does That Look Like for You?

Everyone deals with change differently. Routine makes us feel safe because our lives are ever so slightly predictable with a routine in place. Changing something – even if it's just changing our mind about a certain activity– disrupts this routine.

For some people, that can lead to stress and negative emotions. Some become angry at the new activity for disrupting the routine.

Others blame themselves, thinking that if they weren't so incompetent, they'd be able to keep their old routine. Some start trying to blame everything and everyone around them. It is very difficult for many of us to accept change for what it is: something different.

This can be especially compounded when the reason we're making a change in the first place is because we have found ourselves in a bad spot mentally and emotionally. It may feel that nothing will ever be "good" again. We may feel that we deserve to accept a life in which things don't always go smoothly, and we're constantly feeling negative emotions on top of negative emotions because our emotional outbursts can lead to feelings of guilt, panic, depression, anxiety, and more.

And now we're asking our brains to shoulder even more stress as we work to turn things right-side up again. We've already had to confront our emotions and accept the fact that our current patterns aren't helping us achieve the mental and emotional status we desire. We've gone so far as to really examine options that can help us reach our goals. Now we must put a plan in place to help us make a change, and that can be very, very intimidating. That's what makes the preparation stage of change so important for many people.

There are the types of people who prefer drastic changes. You've likely heard phrases like "quitting cold turkey," "close the deal," or "rip off the bandage." Much like a diver plunging into icy-cold waters from a terrifying height, these folks prefer to jump right into something, absorb the shock, and proceed as quickly as possible. The rationale behind this theory is that getting change over with quickly will make it easier to deal with the pain of change. Just yanking off an adhesive bandage as rapidly as possible will hurt more at first, but the painful stage will be over more quickly than if you slowly work the bandage off.

This method doesn't work for everyone. Just as ripping off a bandage quickly can cause more damage to different types of skin, applying change immediately isn't a good method for everyone's mental state. If you are the type of person who can take a plunge and stick with it, I commend you!

Other types of people prefer to make changes slowly. They know that, for them, change can be a difficult process, and enacting change without a clear path and strong support system is more likely to result in abandoning the whole project.

I'd like to take a moment to note that abandoning change is not failure. This is not a pass-fail scenario. As one of my mentors once explained to me, "the behavioral change wagon moves very slowly, so if you fall off, you just have to dust yourself off and get yourself back on it." While you don't want to accept failure before you even start, now is a good time to set the expectation that this might not be easy, and you might experience varying degrees of success throughout the process.

So how do we prepare for change? This can be different for each individual. Some people like to create a schedule for how they'll incorporate new behaviors within the context of each day. The first day, they might complete one beneficial activity then continue to increasingly replace the old routine with the new one until the new activity has become the regular routine.

But for those of us who are working on unpredictable behaviors associated with mental and emotional health, it's not quite that simple. We may not know when we're going to be triggered, or when trauma is going to rear its ugly head, encouraging us to behave in a way that makes no sense to us. Most of us do not experience the same emotional triggers every single day, which means we may not be able to make small, gradual transitions over a long period of time.

Instead, consider taking a step in the new direction each time you feel your mental health threatened. We don't always get the benefit of knowing that we're about to reach a highly emotional state before we get there, but when you feel things moving around in your mental status, you might start contemplating your new activity before things get chaotic.

Another one of my mentors once explained, "in order to make change happen, we need to accept that change happens in the first place." One way we can do that is to make less stressful changes before making big ones.

Mini- Activity: How to Incorporate Small Changes into Your Day

It may seem counter-intuitive, but one of the best ways to make big changes is to try out different little changes. Sometimes, if we start switching things around on ourselves regularly, our brain will let go of the notion that routine is "safe," and allow more opportunities to occur.

What does your routine look like now? Is it highly regimented, or is the only pattern in your life the complete lack of organization? Many of us fall somewhere in between the two. We wake up at a certain time most days. We shower, eat breakfast, and brush our teeth in a specific order. We complete our daily tasks, have meals around the same time each day, and generally do the same things in the evening. You might be surprised to discover that even the most spontaneous days have a lot of routine to them.

Example:
Travis is a freelance artist who travels the country in his van. He's rarely in the same place for more than a week, and he's always trying out new things.

However, he finds that he wakes up naturally around 7am most days. He likes to start the day off with coffee and yoga after walking his dog. He typically has a sandwich around noon. Even though he's always in a different location, he's a little surprised to note that he spends most of his days either driving or working on his art, and most nights are spent at open mic nights in the various towns in which he stops throughout his travels.

Routines often happen when we're least suspecting it, and everything from our emotional patterns to physical patterns are impacted by change.

Therefore, some people like to shake things up a little bit before making big changes to lessen the impact to their routine.

Here are some things to ask yourself:
- What time do I typically start my day?
- What activities do I do first?
- How attached am I to my routine?

- How do I feel when things change (e.g.- an appointment in the middle of the day)?
- Are there parts of my day that are not as regimented, and if so, how do I spend that time?
- What would happen if I did something out of the ordinary?

You may wish to pay special attention to what you do over the course of a few days to really get a grip on how your routine works for you.

Then, change something small. Perhaps you drive a specific route to school or work– try a different way. Maybe you always order the same sandwich from the same cafe– choose a different sandwich. From wearing socks you normally wouldn't choose to taking the stairs when you'd normally take the elevator, try to do something just a little different to shake things up. Your goal is to change things just enough that you're no longer on your previous routine, but still accomplishing the same tasks each day.

Remember, you're not trying to disrupt everything with massive changes, unless you feel that making a significant change is a very comfortable and logical step. Instead, the goal is to convince yourself that moving away from your regular routine will still be safe and reasonable.

If you find that these little changes are disrupting your day too much, it might be time to back off a bit. Minimize the changes until they are no longer uncomfortable. Everyone will take a different amount of time to become accustomed to the idea of change, so there's no need to rush through or set a harsh schedule for yourself.

As you do, keep track of how you feel about all of this. Even if you don't really notice a difference in your emotional or mental state, that's worth noting. You might find that something you thought would be significant, such as trying a different route for your commute, was enjoyable, whereas something that you thought you wouldn't notice, such as wearing different socks, created a significant difference in your approach to the day. In fact, many people find that keeping track of how small changes impact their mental and emotional health makes them more in tune with their overall wellbeing. By tracking your reactions to minor events, you may eventually find that you have a better understanding of why major events impact you in more negative ways.

Putting your emotional and mental health together is a series of mindfulness exercises, and by helping you get into the right mindset for change, you may discover a few things about why your triggers and trauma impact you the way they do.

What Challenges Do You Expect to Encounter?

Another way to prepare yourself for change is to carefully consider the challenges you may encounter along the way. For some individuals, it helps to set expectations before embarking on any type of new activity.

There is the risk that you can create what is known as a "self-fulfilling prophecy" by doing this, so it's important to approach this strategy carefully. First, we need to understand clearly what a self-fulfilling prophecy really is.

The term itself is relatively new. Robert K. Merton first used the term self-fulfilling prophecy in 1948 in an article published in *The Antioch Review* to describe "a false definition of the situation evoking a behavior which makes the originally false conception come true". Essentially, you think you're going to mess things up in a specific way to the point where your fears become a prediction.

There is a fine line between expecting challenges and refusing to accept success. Many people– especially those with various types of mental illness that are related to anxiety diagnoses– can find an endless array of things that can go wrong in any new experience. I speak as someone who has invented all sorts of disasters when change is in the air. However, I have learned that sometimes thinking about what realistically could "go wrong" can be comforting.

This book is all about exploring the challenges that occur when our emotional and mental health isn't acceptable to us. We have investigated several exercises that are intended to bring us closer to consciously understanding and maintaining our emotional reactions to stressors. While we are looking to create change in our physical behavior or psychological state, we are becoming more mindful of what our emotions are and are creating a more conscious relationship between our conscious and emotional mind. Our conscious mind can make choices, whereas our emotional mind works on autopilot, rarely without our conscious input.

Connecting with difficult topics, like what challenges we might expect when enacting change, can give us a different glimpse into our emotional mind. Many times, what we perceive as challenges are our own anxieties and fear of failure bubbling to the surface.

As you consider what challenges you might encounter when adding more mindful activities to your mental health toolbox, let yourself explore why that challenge exists. Some might be obviously connected to trauma you have experienced. If this is the case, re-examine the activity itself. You do not need to replace something that is not working with something that is destined to fail. This is about as reasonable as replacing a tire with a slow leak with one that is completely flat.

Many of us have the temptation to make change as uncomfortable as possible for ourselves. Resist this urge! Discovering that your current patterns aren't working isn't a bad thing. It is an amazing opportunity to reconnect with yourself and discover how you can learn to heal and grow. Sure, it feels crummy and uncomfortable and brings with it a whole new world of emotions to deal with, but you are giving yourself the opportunity to try something new instead of continuing with your current state of suffering.

You may wish to write down your challenges so you can really sit with them for a while to absorb the root of this challenge. You may prefer not to write anything down, so you don't have to obsess over a truth you might not be ready to confront. Either method is fine if you allow yourself to appreciate why change is uncomfortable for you, and how you can address each potential challenge as it arises– *if* it arises!

> *Example:*
> *After I decided I didn't want to take part in the daily office cheese party, I felt like I was isolating myself from my coworkers. I felt like they thought I was trying to be "better" than them by not eating my emotions. I really wasn't thinking about them– I wanted to make this change for myself.*

As a result, I started feeling anxious any time I was speaking with my coworkers. Were they thinking that I was being condescending? Did they not want to hang out with me? I became paranoid that my coworkers didn't like me anymore.

In reality, I was projecting my own feelings of negative self-worth onto my coworkers. When I spoke to them about my fears, they confirmed that they really hadn't thought anything of my lack of participation in the cheese buffet. They assumed I was making a choice that was important for me and that it had nothing to do with our work relationships.

I wasn't afraid of change because I wanted cheese– I was afraid that I would be lonely and ostracized. Those feelings were based on my own trauma, however, and not on the reality of my relationship with my coworkers.

Contemplating challenges may seem like a recipe for disaster, and it can wade into self-fulfilling prophecy territory if left unchecked. However, if you truly consider the challenges you expect, you may find yourself learning a bit more about your true emotional state.

What Will You Do When That Happens?

One significant benefit of considering the challenges you may encounter as you work to stabilize and connect with your emotional and mental phases is that you can create a game plan. You can think to yourself, "If ___ happens, I will do ___."

When things don't go the way we planned, many of us fall into emotional disarray. We have failed, we are lousy, we are terrible, we don't deserve good things, etc. We may feel we're selfish for wanting to improve our lifestyle or that we are being narcissistic for focusing on our own needs. Failure is an apt punishment for such sins, right?

Wrong. The word "failure" implies that there is no opportunity to do anything about the results of your experiment.

> *Example:*
> *Clancy tried getting up at 5am to do yoga in order to give them a good rush of natural endorphins before facing a rocky day of school. After three days, they stopped getting up so early and zipped through a few half-hearted stretches. They noticed that they did not feel the same as when they did a complete yoga session, but the extra sleep felt good.*
>
> *Clancy believes they have chosen a poor activity and is grumpy that it "didn't work." However, Clancy still truly enjoys yoga and how they feel even after a 20-minute session.*

Things rarely go according to plan, which is why we develop strategies and contingencies. Doing this for your change process can help you be prepared when things don't work out exactly as you expected.

Clancy is not alone in craving those extra minutes of sleep, but there are many opportunities in their scenario. Perhaps they schedule yoga for a different time of day. Maybe they shorten their morning practice so they can get the best of both worlds. Change within change is uncomfortable for many people, but if you allow yourself to mindfully plan for these road bumps, you may be able to navigate them more successfully.

Remind yourself as many times as you need to that changing your routine as well as adding and subtracting activities from your life is not a binding contract. Even if you are not a flexible person by nature, there is flexibility in the choices you make. Each choice you make has its own unique set of benefits and consequences.

Acknowledging the challenges you may experience as you attempt to enact change brings you closer to understanding why these challenges exist, but in the meantime, consider carefully how you will meet these challenges. Often, we immediately become emotional when things don't go the way we expected them to go. Disappointment, despair, longing, anger, blame, frustration, guilt, and sadness are all common emotional responses to things not working out as planned, but all emotions are valid.

Change is hard because change generates emotion. We experience hopes, fears, determination, and defeat. Every day is different, and the solace we found in our existing routine is shaken. Nothing is the same as it was, and we may feel completely thrown off in all areas of our life, even if the change we're trying to enact looks like it should be insignificant.

There is no "should" when it comes to creating new patterns for your emotional and mental well-being. There are only things that you are doing, can do, or are not doing. Furthermore, you should not judge yourself for what you can do, or what you are or are not doing. Instead, focus on how each step brings you a little closer to your emotional reality, and how each leap forward or set back teaches you something even more interesting about your mental health.

Sometimes as we prepare for change, we need to consider how to best appreciate the myriad of feelings we're experiencing. There can be many methods for tracking your thoughts all of which can help you grow closer to understanding your emotions.

Exercise: Experimenting with Journaling

By nature, I am not a journal-er. I am terrified of writing out my thoughts and making them tangible. I don't fear other people judging me for what I write in my journal; I am terrified of what I will think about what I've written in my journal.

As a writer, I often re-read what I've written several times to make sure it's perfect. My editors are very aware that it's never perfect, and that a perfect manuscript does not exist. But in my mind, I always need to be certain that I'm at least expressing my thoughts correctly, even if the words become jumbled or riddled with typos.

I apply this same logic to journaling, which means I find myself obsessing over a sentence I wrote rather than becoming introspective. "Did I really say that? Do I mean that? Is it okay to feel like that?" This type of behavior is not helpful when working on your mental health.

However, there are some times when even anxious perfectionists like myself agree it can be helpful to experiment with journaling. Periods of change are often a fantastic time to do some form of self-reflection to make sure your conscious and emotional mind are in agreement. If not, this is also a great exercise for helping to realign your thoughts and emotions.

So, what's a good way for people who don't like to journal to feel comfortable journaling? Let's look at a few different ways to really track our emotions and understand what we're feeling along with how and why we're experiencing such complicated emotions.

Option 1: Prompt Journaling

Some folks do their best work when they have some specific direction to work with. Prompt journaling involves selecting a specific topic to reflect upon throughout the journal entry. Prompts can range from very precise such as "what is really upsetting me right now?" to very broad subjects such as "how do you think you've changed in the past ten years?"

Prompt journaling helps us focus our thoughts when we sit down to write. Oftentimes, we can be so overwhelmed by whatever is happening in our lives that what we write reflects our emotional state but doesn't tell us much about our mental state. You've probably experienced this type of "word salad" when someone asks you to describe how you feel in the heat of an emotional moment. Sometimes the words don't make sense. You might yell or write in all capital letters, bold font and underlining absolutely everything so that you can appropriately express ***how very strongly you are feeling these emotions!!!!!!***

Having a prompt can help organize and direct these feelings so that instead of ranting and raving, you are having a productive conversation with your own brain. Answering a question requires more focus than simply "writing about how you feel."

I've created a collection of some journal prompts that I have found helpful in the Resources section at the end of this book to get you started. Your mental health care providers may also have some excellent prompts suited perfectly for your individual situation as well.

Option 2: Handwriting Your Journal
Yes, this is the 21st century, and there are dozens of ways technology has come to make journaling easier. You can type, voice memo, blog, vlog, or express your emotions on one or all of a myriad of social media outlets.

For the sake of really connecting with your mental and emotional state, consider handwriting a few journal entries. Note how the experience is different from any other format you have used for journaling. Does it feel more personal or impersonal? Do you dig deeper into your emotions and current events when you type, record, or hand write your entries?

Another consideration for handwriting your journal is that it is completely in your hands what you choose to do with your results. You are not forced to save it on a cloud or a drive. You don't have to "publish" or "make private." You don't have to fit a specific time slot, dress a certain way, or carefully consider the soundtrack. Once you've wrapped up an entry, you can save it, rip it into tiny bits, burn it (safely), or share it with your support team. If words fail you, you can use drawings to express your thoughts. A private journal is yours and yours alone, and no one has to know you ever had a handwritten journal but you.

As a result, some people feel very comfortable with this method over others because it allows them to be completely honest without fear of judgment from others. In fact, I prefer this method because I know I won't go back to try to edit– first, I would have to decipher my chicken scratches!

Option 3: Choosing a Journal App

And for those on the other side of the analog/tech debate, there are many quality options available for journaling apps.

Today's apps offer much more than a clean space for you to dutifully type your thoughts and feelings. Some offer the ability to log moods and events with time stamps that can help you search for particular days. Some allow users to set goals and track progress, which can be very helpful for those who are looking for additional accountability in making changes in their lives. Some even offer therapeutic services such as prompts based on specific behaviors or activities to help with calming and redirecting/reframing negative thoughts.

The concept of an interactive journal is relatively new, so you may experience some "growing pains" when trying out a new platform. Bear in mind that some of these apps have a monthly or annual cost associated with them, so it's not a bad idea to do a little extra research to make sure you're investing in the best option for your needs. I have included a list of some popular journaling apps in the Resources section to get you started.

Option 4: Making Time

Another technique that some folks use to keep them on track with their journaling involves scheduling a specific time for the activity. If you have chosen a new activity that involves updating your daily schedule, you may wish to add in some time for journaling as part of your mindfulness and wellness routine.

Choosing to journal at a very specific time each day can be helpful for several reasons. First, some people feel that having a deadline for various activities makes them feel more accountable. If they know when they should be doing something, they show up and engage in that activity at that set time. Setting aside time for this activity also allows some individuals to get into the mind frame they need to be in when trying to express and process their emotions and overall mental health.

Of all the options presented here, this one can be the most polarizing as some people feel that being "forced" to write at a specific time inspires more negative emotions. If you are one of these people, do not try to make yourself journal each day at 4pm on the dot. Even if you think it would be the "best thing" to help with accountability, you are already enacting enough change in your life without finding a new way to resent your choices. Being strict with yourself is not conducive to understanding and forgiving yourself which are two of the important factors that will help you make change happen in the first place.

If you have discovered you are not, by nature, a journal-er, consider using one of these options to help you record, reflect, and reminisce about your journey through emotional mindfulness.

Is journaling absolutely necessary? Of course not! Just like every other aspect of your mental health journey, everything you do should be carefully considered based on expert advice. And as you are your own best expert, that means you get to choose what activities you complete. You choose your own adventure through connecting with your emotions, adding tools to your coping toolbox, and observing what that does for you.

Sometimes it feels like our mental and emotional health voyage is less of a well-mapped trip and more like a maze. Sometimes we think we're on the right path, only to turn a corner into a dead end. We may double back on our steps or stand in one spot for a few extra moments while we try to figure things out. Often, we get a little lost, and that can bring about a new set of challenging emotions and mental health triggers.

The maze you are about to enter may seem overwhelming, but it is safe if you let it be safe. You always have an option to reach out to your care team, including trusted friends and family members as well as your preferred mental health professionals. You are not doing it wrong as long as you are doing something, even if that "something" is not moving for a second while you analyze a situation in detail.

This is not a race or a competition. The only "prize" waiting at the end is the knowledge that you can continue to grow as a person.

That also means that change will not "fix" you. As we move towards the actual change process, take time to remind yourself that the goal is not to eliminate your emotions because that is currently impossible. Instead, it's to understand them, connect with them, and appreciate what causes them so that you can express them in a healthy way.

At this stage, you now have a metaphorical box of nice new shiny toys, and you're about to try them out for the first time. The preparation stage is all about seeing how those tools feel and whether you think they're right for the job at hand. Now, it's time to see how well they work!

CHANGING THE WORLD – OR AT LEAST, YOUR OWN WORLD

If you're hoping this is the part of the book where I divulge the magical secrets of how to change your mind, get a grip on your emotions, and start acting like a "normal" person starting tomorrow morning, I'm afraid you've come a long way towards disappointment.

Science doesn't fully understand emotions, just as we have a tenuous grasp on why some individuals are more prone to mental illness than others. We don't know why some people "just get over it" while others are psychologically devastated by the same event. There is no logic; therefore, we can't target the exact problem to "fix" it.

What we're learning instead is that there is no "normal." Even though we all inhabit this planet in a similar body, the electrified Jell-O that calls the shots doesn't work the same in every single body. Is it nature or nurture? How do siblings process identical trauma differently? Why does the same nervous system that courses through each of our bodies fail to operate with identical results in different individuals?

Simply put: we don't know. Psychology and psychiatry, as we currently recognize them, are fairly new sciences. Gone are the days when we attempted to make diagnoses based on skull bumps or threw tokens to read the humors. But from these failed attempts at understanding the human brain and "what makes us tick" we've gained a deeper appreciation of how truly mysterious the brain is.

As much as I would love to tell you that everything will go beautifully and you'll be a completely changed and emotionally balanced person in just seven days, I can't. There are no guarantees in mental and emotional health journeys, but there is one trend that nearly all scientists can agree on: doing nothing does, quite literally, nothing. Nothing will change if you do not proceed with making the change happen.

When you look at what you're about to do on paper, it may look pretty "easy" and reasonable to you: "So when I get triggered, I think about petting my dog or actually pet my dog, and then I feel all better?" What we're doing in this book could technically be simplified to that level, but it's a little more involved than petting your dog when you're mad. Consider reframing the process like this: "So when I get triggered, I acknowledge my emotions, but I focus on my coping tools instead of having an emotional outburst. This allows me to become more in tune with what is truly causing my emotions and helps me deal with the emotions in a way that is not harmful to myself or others."

So, which is the reality? Is it as simple as petting the dog more, or is it as complicated as being aware of every type of emotion you're feeling at any given time and immediately connecting it with a soothing activity or coping mechanism? The answer, of course, is "both."

Over time, mindfully experiencing your emotions will allow you to be more aware of them and their impact on your life. You'll eventually be able to consciously explore your feelings and tap into their origins and what impact they've had on your life so far. But that is a very long-term goal that starts with this act of mindfulness.

The stage that we are currently addressing is the start of this process. You are beginning the journey of connecting with your mental health and emotional reactions. You are working to understand which emotions are evoked at which time. You have gathered the tools needed to help you process emotions in a helpful, healthful way, and you are prepared to start consciously using those tools. Now, it is time to apply what you've learned about yourself to your daily life.

However, many people find that change stirs up a lot of emotions not just about the change process itself, but about prior behaviors. As things get better, we often realize how "bad" they really were in the first place. Let's look at some of the typical emotional responses to change and how to keep forward momentum through some of the negative emotions we might feel as we find new balance in our lives.

Getting over the Guilt

One of my mentors once said, "guilt should have its own ICD-10 code," because of how prevalent it is among those of us who live with mental illness. Not only are we made to feel somehow "less than" neurotypical individuals, but we're often held to a higher level of accountability for our emotional reactions. Many of us have had family, friends, and even complete strangers offer unkind words about how we behave when triggered or processing trauma. We can be accused of attention seeking, narcissism, and being ungrateful, among other generalizations that are made about behavior that others simply do not understand.

Indeed, there is nothing "normal" about experiencing mental illness which is why many of us have a hard time coping with our emotions in the first place. Compounded with the harsh words of those around us, we often feel guilty for acting "the way we do." Being told "you shouldn't act like that" or "stop being like that" can be extremely traumatic for those of us who are trying the best we can with the brains and bodies we've been given.

This guilt can move its way to center stage when we start performing activities or adopt behaviors that stand in stark contrast to our typical state of being. People may notice that you are "getting better" and compliment you on the changes you've made. While these are often meant as kind words, they can be seriously traumatic to the individuals during a change.

I like to think of my life, my actions, my attitude, and my emotions as a "working draft." I'm constantly editing and changing things. And while I can't change the past, I can look at the parts that I don't like very much as something to move away from with the actions I take today. My previous meltdowns are recorded forever in history, but the way I react to similar situations today determines my future. My future self has the potential to be much stronger than the version of myself who had no toolbox, let alone tools. There is hope, and hope can be much stronger than regret.

For some individuals, the guilt associated with prior behaviors can be overwhelming, especially when other people in our lives enjoy reminding us of, "that one time when... ." We cannot expect anyone to forget the past incidents that impacted them, least of all ourselves. How many nights have you stayed up long past your bedtime, sliding down the sneaky hate spiral inspired by all the hateful, unnecessary things you've done in your life? This emotional response, though terrible, is pretty common.

First, it's important to cut yourself and others off about the past. Try to say– to yourself or anyone else who brings up these events– "I'm very sorry for what happened then. I don't want to revisit it right now because I am using my energy to focus on a brighter future." Don't ignore or deny, but also don't allow that hate spiral to unfold in front of you.

You may need to pull out some of the coping tools and activities from your collection when guilt starts to creep up on you. Guilt can be a very overwhelming emotion, and brings with it sadness, anger, confusion, and other negative feelings. The tools we brainstormed earlier can be used any time emotions run high, not just when you are feeling triggered by a specific scenario. Guilt is an emotion, too, and in order to help us understand our emotions, we need to connect with all our emotions, not just the ones we're most familiar with.

You may wish to diagram your feelings of guilt, as we did in the first exercise. Identifying the different emotional aspects of your guilt can help you realize why you're feeling this way, which in turn can help you pull out just the right tool to help you process and move forward through it.

Guilt is a natural emotional reaction for those who are working towards making important changes in their lives. Even if the activity you are using to help you consciously connect with your emotions is something regular and unobtrusive– such as playing with your pet– it is possible to have thoughts like "I should have done this long ago," or "my life would be so much better if I had tried this sooner." Those intrusive thoughts aren't technically incorrect, but they don't take into consideration all the steps you have taken just to make a little change that has a huge impact on your emotional and mental health.

Appreciate and Accept

In addition to processing the guilt associated with your past and present emotional reactions, it can be very helpful to pause, appreciate, and accept the path that you are on.

On one hand, looking at how far you have come with pride and hope for the future is very rewarding. If you kept your mood maps from the first exercise as well as any journal notes throughout the process, you can likely track your progress. You may become emotional looking at all of the challenges you have overcome and how much more connected you are to your emotional state now. You may be thrilled that you are more understanding of your triggers and how you can intelligently connect to your emotions to prevent harmful behaviors.

But those emotions are usually only this easily accessible on "good" days. When we're having less than stellar days– physically, psychologically, emotionally, or all the above– we can easily become trapped by the pressing fear that we are not doing enough.

Sometimes others in our lives say or do something that makes us feel like we're not working at all. We may feel like we're not doing enough, working hard enough, or making enough progress. Even worse, because change is not a linear process, and emotions are unpredictable, there is not a standard of measurement for progress. You may feel very triumphant one day, only to experience very negative emotions the next. When we and those around us recognize only the bad days without giving proper credit to process, it can be very tempting to just give up.

As difficult as it may be, it is important to acknowledge that you are on an amazing journey. Success is not guaranteed. Even on days when you give your best effort towards connecting with your emotional support tools and mental health journey, it doesn't take too much of a disruption to cause complete chaos.

Though you may find yourself easily sliding into previous habits during highly stressful times, that doesn't mean you've failed, or that you must start over from the beginning again. To add insult to injury, this sensation of failure can increase the volatility of an emotional breakdown, slamming the door in the face of any logic or tools that might be available to intercept your unchecked emotions.

Your emotional responses may have created problems in the past, and they may continue to do so. Individuals from all backgrounds and mental health statuses are prone to becoming overwhelmed by emotion and lashing out in ways that may seem illogical. You are not the only person who has been in this situation. You are not the only person who lives with the impact, complications, and challenges created by emotional reactions. You are not the only person who struggles with their mental health. You are not the only person who has trauma or is triggered by things that others might find "silly." You are a person trying their best to do their best with everything that this brand-new day has laid before you.

There may be days when tears well up in your eyes and you easily– almost automatically– take a few deep breaths, put your finger directly on what triggered you, complete your coping activity, manage to find a place where you can think logically about the emotions you are feeling, and talk yourself through the situation to a state of inner peace. There may also be days when you are unable to connect with any of the activities on your list, and you honestly believe that you will never feel better ever again.

So, why do we bother? Why even try to connect with our mental and emotional health, if we're never going to have perfect success in controlling our emotions?

Progress is not linear. Businesses, crops, the stock market, your favorite sports team, and you will all experience ups and downs over time. As of the publishing date of this book, there is no method that will simply stop negative feelings, overwhelming emotions, or the effects of mental illness. As the saying goes, there are good days and bad days. However, one of my coaching colleagues once made a good point about how mindfulness works, "If you're currently having a lot of bad days, it stands to reason that any change you make has a really good chance of making the opposite true." That is to say that if you are currently dissatisfied with your day-to-day emotional and mental state, it is more likely that any change you make will have a positive impact, rather than a negative one.

Let go of the concept of "success vs. failure" in this instance and participate in the adventure of rediscovering yourself. That's much easier said than done, but it is a compromise you will need to make with any glimmer of perfectionism you may notice. If your goal is to connect with your emotional self to make positive changes in your mental health, then you will need to recognize that there will be many bumps in the road. You will likely learn things about yourself that you aren't able to connect with right away. The phrase "warts and all" comes to mind, as when you start unveiling your emotional status to yourself, you often find some trauma, triggers, and intrusive thoughts that have been lying dormant for some time.

As I've mentioned several times, I strongly encourage you to take this journey with a strong support team. That includes professionals, such as a psychiatrist, therapist, or primary care physician, as well as individuals you trust on a personal level. You will need to explain how much and in what way you want them to participate in your journey, so it's a good idea to choose friends and family members who you trust.

If you are a private individual, you may not wish to "advertise" what you're going through. It is understandable that you might not want everyone trying to butt into your journey and ask questions all the time. It's also normal to let feelings like shame or fear of failure prevent you from communicating your plans with others. Knowing who to trust can also be difficult, especially if you are currently in a new, raw emotional state.

There are resources available for those who are interested in anonymous or semi-private forums for sharing your personal struggles. I have included a few outlets that provide support to users in the Resources section of this book.

While you may wish to "go at it alone," it can be very helpful to have your support team fully updated and ready to be by your side as you work to connect with your mental health and express your emotions in a more positive way.

You may encounter someone who voices an opinion along the lines of, "well, I don't think you deserve to be happy, given the way you treated me in the past!" In order to move forward, you will need to accept and appreciate the consequences of your past actions. That means acknowledging that what you did had an impact on someone else's well-being and apologizing for how your actions or reactions have continued to resonate with that individual. However, your ownership of your actions ends at admitting fault and taking accountability.

Unfortunately, in many emotional encounters with other individuals, there are multiple versions of what happened: their version, your version, a passerby's version, a friend's version, the version that got passed through rumor mills, and so forth. That's why it can be beneficial to be specific in your admissions.

Example:
Ryan and Rick are siblings. Years ago, Ryan said some hateful things to Rick in the heat of an argument. Rick was traumatized by the things Ryan said, and his own reaction caused him to

make decisions he now regrets. As a result of these decisions, Rick lost his job and broke up with his partner.

Rick holds Ryan responsible for the loss of his job and partner. Ryan feels a lot of guilt about what he said back then. However, in working with his therapist, he has come to realize that while he is responsible for saying horrible things, he did not cause Rick to make the decisions he made. To acknowledge the role he has played in Rick's life, Ryan could say something like:

I am sorry for the things I said to you. It was not appropriate for me to say hateful things. I understand that my actions have had a negative impact on your wellbeing, and for that I am sorry.

Notice that in this example, Ryan is not accepting accountability for Rick's decision making. That's because while his actions impacted Rick's choices, he cannot be responsible for Rick's reaction. It is simply not possible or even logical to accept the blame for the choices someone made in reaction to their own triggers. If that were the case, then no one would ever have to appreciate and accept any of their own actions, as nearly everything we say or do is in relation to something said or done by someone else!

Everyone's words and actions matter. Intent is not magical. As humans, we will both experience and inspire a full range of emotions. Whether our emotions are a personal reaction or meant to be shared, they are honest reflections of our mental and physical status during intense stimulation. Misunderstandings occur, and people will take things personally when you may not have even intended for them to observe these actions and reactions. Be sure to carefully consider the authentic impact of your action, and don't blindly accept the blame others may pass on to you as you are working to heal your previous wounds and grow as an individual.

As you continue your path to better mental health and understanding of your emotions, there will be many standout moments where you will need to appreciate and accept what is happening, even if it isn't exactly where you had hoped, planned, or expected to be. You may not believe yourself at first but affirming to yourself that you do appreciate and accept what you are doing and what you hope to achieve can be validating, especially on days when you're feeling challenged.

Here are a few phrases you may wish to add to your toolbox. You may wish to repeat these statements out loud or to yourself or incorporate them in your journal entries:

- I appreciate and accept that I have chosen to make a change in my life.
- I appreciate and accept that changing my relationship with my emotions may be difficult.
- I appreciate and accept that some days will be more challenging than others.
- I appreciate and accept that I may take steps forward and backward – healing is not a linear process.
- I appreciate and accept the assistance provided to me by my support team.

, appreciate and accept my decision to connect more with my emotional states.

- I appreciate and accept that mental wellness is not a static condition, and that I may experience setbacks.
- I appreciate and accept that I am undergoing a process that may uncover more truths about myself, which can be uncomfortable to process.
- I appreciate and accept the role that I may have played in someone else's trauma.

Over time, you may come to realize that you do, in fact, appreciate and accept this process. While mental illness and being emotionally overwhelmed hardly meet the traditional definition of "enjoyment," it is possible that the steps you take on your journey will make you feel empowered to continue taking more and more steps towards a more mindful future.

Inspiration, Not Obsession

Another common pratfall experienced by those who are trying to make significant changes in their lives is the fear of doing anything but what you believe you should be doing. It is not uncommon for folks to become obsessed with a particular activity that is helping them and cling to it for safety.

There can be various stages and levels of obsession. Some people feel that if they can't do things exactly according to their prescribed routine, something terrible will happen. We discussed self-fulfilling prophecies earlier, and this type of instinct falls under that category. One of the wonderful things about our mental health toolbox is that, unlike an actual toolbox, it does not become heavier or bigger as we add more tools to it. That means it is extremely portable and can be taken absolutely anywhere with you.

When you find yourself in an emotional state and you can't play with your dog, or light a candle and take a bath, or play a game of chess immediately, don't panic. Panic rarely helps bring clarity to an already emotional situation. Instead, scour through your mental health toolbox to find something you can do right now.

At first, this might be difficult as you have taught yourself how to automatically reach for the same tool every time you've found yourself experiencing emotional or mental health issues. I personally have spent many cumulative hours in a bathroom, my car, or any other private place, trying desperately to figure out what I can do to work my way out of feeling so awful.

When this happens, it may be helpful to isolate yourself from others, especially if your emotional reaction causes you to act violently or have a very passionate outburst. If you feel that you are on the precipice of harming yourself, however, that may not be the best idea. You may wish to reach out to a member of your medical or personal support team to help you through this moment.

Whether you're alone in the office bathroom or on the phone with your best friend, the next step is to discover the trigger to this incident. Sometimes that's easy, and other times, your emotional state is brought about by a whole series of events that have been leaning on your mental wellness over the course of hours, days, or even weeks. Take the time to question and analyze your emotional state. If you have the ability to draw out a diagram like we did in our first exercise, this can be helpful, but it's okay if you are not capable of that much thinking in the heat of the moment. Instead, consider what was said or done by whom and how it relates to your triggers.

Next, ask yourself what you can do right now. Most likely, your thoughts and emotions are going to be swirling around like a hurricane, preventing you from grasping at any logical thought. As you mindfully breathe, ask yourself as many times as you need to "what can I do right now?" Eventually, you will get an answer. Don't force it.

Some people prefer to ask themselves "what do I want right now?" and you certainly may do so, if it helps. For others– myself included– the answer to that question is often riddled with violent and permanent solutions, so reframing it in terms of being capable of doing something, rather than desiring it, can be helpful in that case.

Once you know what you are capable of, start connecting each forward step to your mindfulness activities. Maybe all you can do is sit on the floor and cry now, but when you're done, maybe you could look forward to splashing some cold water on your face and making a cup of tea. Perhaps you need to sit in your car and scream for the next few minutes, but what's something from your list of activities that you could do after that? When do you think you'll be able to get back on target with your activity? What's a good substitute for that right now?

Often, this type of forward-looking will help us get past the fact that we can't ride out our emotions according to the prescription we wrote for ourselves earlier in this book. That's why we came up with as many different options as possible when brainstorming. There may come a time when we can't do exactly what we want to do to quell our mental and emotional pain, so that means finding another tool to use that will do the trick.

It may be that the tool we try at first doesn't do the trick. Just as an experienced carpenter will keep looking for the right tool, so too can you continuously revisit your toolbox. Sure, it's not an instant fix, but little in the mental health/emotional wellness world is. A carpenter could slap some duct tape on your broken door and call it good enough, but we all know that mending and reframing things takes time and effort. That's why we try and try again to find mindfulness in our worst moments of emotional and mental illness.

Other types of obsessions go the other direction. Sometimes we feel like we can't do anything except the behavior we deem safe. Obsessive compulsive disorder (OCD) is currently considered an anxiety disorder and includes the ritualization of certain behaviors or actions. However, this isn't the only condition associated with relying exclusively on one or more activities in order to cope with emotional and mental strife.

Earlier, I mentioned that routine often provides us with a sense of security. Sometimes, it takes a small leap for our brain to decide that the safety of routine is the only way to be safe. There is some truth to this– if we don't manifest anything out of the ordinary, it is far less likely that anything surprising will happen– but unfortunately, it's not a reliable way to predict outcomes.

If you have struggled with addictive behaviors in the past, you may wish to work closely with your professional and personal care team regarding the changes you are attempting to make. While there's nothing wrong with approaching a new activity or change with gusto, it's also important that you take care of yourself. If you notice yourself spending more time practicing mindfulness and your coping activities than you do eating, bathing, sleeping, or getting work done, that might be a sign that you are falling into an obsessive pattern.

Because everyone is different, and their relationship with repetitive actions may be the result of various traumas or triggers, there is not a master plan for preventing or disconnecting from obsessive behavior. Avoidance is a method that works for many people– doing things such as deleting an app, getting rid of the video game console, or getting rid of any binge-worthy food are a few examples– but that's often the same quality of "fix" as the carpenter with the duct tape.

You could find a new behavior to expand your toolbox, but often the fear of failure or discomfort will either prohibit you from moving forward, or simply be the gateway to another level of obsession.

That doesn't mean that nothing will help you in this situation. It just means that this type of situation is best left to highly trained professionals, not the kindly mental health folks writing a book of helpful hints. I know from my own lifetime of experience that anxiety can manifest itself in strange ways. When we're attempting to find stability, we may cling to anything that looks like we can hold onto it for a while, regardless of how helpful, or not, that thing may be. And when we discover it's best to hold on, letting go of that one thing can be the most difficult part of the process.

I like to frame the concept as "appreciation, not obsession." I appreciate what my coping mechanisms can do for me. I appreciate how much practicing mindfulness has helped me connect with my erratic emotions. I also appreciate that I have many tools that I can use to help me through traumatic times. I appreciate that I may not be able to reach for the same tool each time. I appreciate the options that I have, and I appreciate that I can connect with my mental health in a variety of ways.

I also appreciate that it has taken me over 40 years to do so, so once again, I beg you to not expect instantaneous results.

For most people, the change process works well at first. We have a behavior to avoid, one to substitute, exercises to go through when things get rough, and a conscious connection to what we're doing. But then we get a little lax. We start thinking we've got this whole thing down pat, and it didn't take nearly as long as we thought it would. Good for us.

But then something happens, and it shakes everything up. With our vision of events blurred through the lens of mental illness, it is easy to consider this the end of everything we've tried so hard to make happen. Whether you give up completely and stop trying to be mindful at all or wander away from the activities that were helping, it's easy to think "that didn't work, so I'm going to stop trying."

Please don't. Relapse is an actual stage of change, because it happens to everyone. As I mentioned earlier, the change wagon moves slowly, and if you happen to fall off or get left behind, it's perfectly fine to catch up to it again and start the process over.

Throughout trying to connect with your own mind and emotional reality, you will want to supply yourself with forgiveness, discipline, reassurance, and grace. Let's look at this process through an exercise.

Exercise: The Gift of Grace

The term "grace" can mean something different to many people. The term is usually found in conversations involving spirituality and faith. According to **Merriam-Webster.com**, the word "grace" can mean:

2a: APPROVAL, FAVOR
b: archaic: MERCY, PARDON
c: a special favor: PRIVILEGE
d: disposition to or an act or instance of kindness, courtesy, or clemency
e: a temporary exemption: REPRIEVE

3a: a charming or attractive trait or characteristic
b: a pleasing appearance or effect: CHARM
c: ease and suppleness of movement or bearing

8a: sense of propriety or right
b: the quality or state of being considerate or thoughtful

I included these three definitions because they align most with the sensations you can experience when you give yourself grace through the process of change. Mercy and pardon are large components of forgiveness. Having the opportunity to work on yourself is very much a privilege. You'll also want to be as graceful as you can be as you move through the various experiences that bring you high emotional content. And yes, the process will require you to be gracious with yourself as well.

You may try to convince yourself that this is a direct process. "If I focus on coping activities instead of my emotions, I won't do the things that have gotten me into trouble in the past." If that were true, there would be far fewer professionals in the psychological field, and this book wouldn't be much more than a few sentences in length.

Instead, here's how far you've come:

1. You have identified that your emotional state has become troublesome to yourself or others.
2. You have taken the time to map your emotions so that you can understand what impacts you along with why and how it impacts you.
3. You have come up with a list of activities that can help you cope with your emotions when they run high.
4. You have consciously selected activities that have the potential to help you after researching how they can help you.
5. You have implemented small and major changes in your life to help you connect to your emotional and mental state in a healthful way.
6. You are consciously choosing to connect with and understand your emotions.

7. You have researched what could possibly go wrong so that you can be prepared for setbacks and relapses.

8. You have taken steps to understand how your emotions can impact your life and that of others, and accepted accountability for your actions.

9. You have learned to appreciate and accept your situation, limitations, and how difficult this journey will be.

10. You have assembled a professional and personal care team to help you stay on track.

11. You are doing the very best you can, every step of the way.

Wow! That's a lot! And when you think about it, even when you're actively working on a later stage, like #11, in which you're constantly working to move forward, you're still working on those earlier steps too. Change is a commitment, just like a marriage, a friendship, or a job. Even when things aren't going as smoothly as you'd like, your commitment to this process is still important, and you deserve grace for not breaking that commitment.

However, it's easy to think we're not doing enough, we're not doing it the right way, or it's taking too long... all the negative self-talk we discussed earlier can and will show up at various points on the journey. Let's find a way to give yourself the gift of grace when you need it most.

Objectives:
- Recognize moments when grace is needed most
- Discover how to manifest that grace

What You'll Need:

- A piece of blank paper (scrap paper is fine)
- A writing utensil - or many, if you prefer!
- A safe, quiet place where you can process emotions
- Optional: your favorite craft supplies
- Optional: a support person, animal, or item that brings you comfort
- Optional: a folder in which you can put written exercises for later reference

Here's what you'll do in this exercise:

- You are going to create a physical manifestation of grace. That might be as simple as writing the word "GRACE" on your paper in big, bold letters, or you may wish to create an elaborate gift for yourself. I've seen cross stitch samplers, keychains, magnets, paintings, ceramics, and even cookies with "Grace" written on the icing.
- As you create the grace that you are going to give to yourself, consider the following think points:
    - I forgive myself for...
    - I am getting better at...
    - I can connect with myself more by...
    - I believe in myself and my efforts because...

You may not have all the answers to these statements at first. You may find that it is impossible to forgive yourself, so why bother? Try to keep in mind that you deserve grace. If not from anyone else in this world, you owe it to yourself to stop punishing yourself for what you've done in the past and allow yourself to move forward to a more promising future.

The Purpose of This Exercise:
- By having an actual, tangible grace to give yourself, you have a constant reminder of what you are doing, how difficult it is, and that you deserve the sensation of grace.
- The act of creating this tangible grace while meditating on the meaning of the word will help you connect to the sensation you deserve.

Pointers:
- Keep your grace somewhere meaningful, so you can mentally or physically meditate on it whenever necessary.
- You can have more than one tangible grace.
- The act of creating can be soothing, so take your time making your own version.

As you work on your physical manifestation of grace, ask yourself what would it take to prevent yourself from dwelling on the "bad stuff"? This can range from constantly replaying old memories of times when you let your emotions get the best of you to regret to making mistakes on your journey. What do you need to do to acknowledge and appreciate those thoughts or feelings in order to move forward?

Also consider, "what type of grace do I need today?" Do you need to be more nimble and agile in navigating your mental and emotional health today? Or is today a day where meditating on forgiveness could be very beneficial? Perhaps you even need the grace to admit that this is not your day, things are not okay, and you need rest. All of these are ways you can give yourself the gift of grace.

Once you've completed this exercise, you'll have your own physical version of grace which you can give yourself, hold closely, or meditate on whenever you need it. It may seem a little cheesy, but sometimes physical props can help us understand when we need to be present for ourselves. It's one thing to say you forgive yourself, and another to experience the weightlessness of letting go of the "bad stuff". It is through the gift of grace that this can happen.

As you become more and more comfortable giving yourself grace for your fumbles, setbacks, and bad days, you may not feel as attached to your physical grace prop. When you discover this, it is a cause to celebrate because you have finally managed to incorporate self-awareness and forgiveness into your mental health toolbox.

CONCLUSION

Since maintaining your emotional and mental health is a life-long process, it seems a bit cruel and ironic to have an ending to this book. Many readers often feel a bit lost or betrayed when they come to the end of a book intended to help them with difficult daily processes, so it's okay if you're left wondering "now what?"

While I would love to be the actual Jiminy Cricket character following you around, helping you make wise choices and keeping you on the path of "goodness," that's unfortunately beyond the scope of reality. However, you have this book, the exercises we've tried, and your support partners to help you as you continue your journey.

I have added a Resources section to the end of this book to help you find even more support. This section includes online tools, apps, experts, and forums to help you access every possible outlet. As I've repeatedly emphasized, your toolbox can never be too full. I encourage you to take a few moments to check out some of the resources that speak to you for future use.

I encourage you to revisit the exercises and activities we've discussed whenever things don't feel quite right. Whether that's an emotional or mental health state that calls your attention to the fact that you need to make a change, revisiting some of these activities can help you re-center and gain more insight into what's going on just outside of your consciousness.

Again, I wish I could tell you that mindfulness is the key, and you'll be completely cured of everything that ails you if you practice this book every single day. Unfortunately, that's not the way humans work. Consider this just one of the many tools you have at your disposal.

Additionally, I encourage everyone who struggles with mental health and emotional wellness to work with professionals in addition to pursuing change behaviors on their own. While this book contains tips and exercises, a professional can interact with you to provide answers, advice, and recommendations based on your official diagnosis and current behavior. If you are looking for a professional or team of professionals, I have included a few potential leads for you in the Resources section.

I hope that you can find peace with your emotions and your mental health. I hope that you can connect to those strange, illusive brain chemicals and make sense of why they do what they do, and how they make you, you. I hope that you can constantly recognize the good within yourself as well as your potential to grow as a human. I hope you give yourself grace whenever you need it, and that you take care of yourself always.

Never forget: your emotions are real, but they do not need to have a negative impact on you or those around you. While our lives are made of many forces we cannot control, you can connect to your emotional well-being and create positive change through understanding.

May your journey bring you wisdom and peace!

RESOURCES

A mental health journey never ends. We live in a world where burnout, uncertainty, and unresolved trauma are often compounded by a lack of resources. Finding professional assistance can be difficult with waiting lists for new patients reaching into months, or even years. Furthermore, there are still plenty of people who believe that mental health issues either don't exist or don't require treatment. As a result, many of us do not have adequate access to the resources we need to fully understand, appreciate, and recognize our mental and emotional needs.

None of these resources are intended to take the place of working with a trained mental health professional– in fact, I've included a few links that can help you find assistance online or in person in the "Experts" section. However, since our professional team can't be with us all day and all night, I've often found solace in checking out some of the following resources.

Please note that no one associated with this book has a connection to or receives remuneration from the sites mentioned. These are simply sites that I have chosen based on merit and that provide a wide range of helpful content. I have arranged these resources by category, so feel free to peruse them all, or specifically those that help you find the information and comfort you need right now.

One word of caution when checking out these sites is to be wary of material that is not appropriate for you right now. While I have vetted these sites for providing appropriate and accurate material, I can't predict how you will personally feel about each one. Therefore, I have the following recommendation: read two sentences, and if it does not serve your purpose, close the tab and move on. I know the world and our opinions can be very volatile, and it is not my goal to trigger any negative emotional response from the folks reading this book. I have provided a brief description of the contents of each site to help mitigate this type of situation.

I hope that this book and some of the resources offered here help you progress in your mental health and emotional wellness journey!

Please note: If you are currently in crisis, please consider this list of resources that can help you immediately, as published by BetterHealth:

Emergency: 911
Suicide & Crisis Lifeline: 988
National Domestic Violence Hotline: 1-800-799-7233
National Hopeline Network: 1-800-SUICIDE (800-784-2433)
Crisis Text Line: Text "DESERVE" TO 741-741
Lifeline Crisis Chat (Online live messaging):
https://suicidepreventionlifeline.org/chat/
Self-Harm Hotline: 1-800-DONT CUT (1-800-366-8288)
Essential local and community services: 211, https://www.211.org/
Planned Parenthood Hotline: 1-800-230-PLAN (7526)
American Association of Poison Control Centers: 1-800-222-1222

National Council on Alcoholism & Drug Dependency Hope Line: 1-800-622-2255

National Crisis Line - Anorexia and Bulimia: 1-800-233-4357

GLBT Hotline: 1-888-843-4564

TREVOR Crisis Hotline: 1-866-488-7386

AIDS Crisis Line: 1-800-221-7044

Veterans Crisis Line: https://www.veteranscrisisline.net

TransLifeline: https://www.translifeline.org - 1-877-565-8860

Experts

This section provides links to a variety of online counseling or therapy options. The relationship between you and your therapist is very personal, so I cannot guarantee that you are going to find a perfect match right away. However, each of these sites comes highly recommended by professionals in the field of psychology, psychiatry, and therapy.

There may be a cost associated with some of these resources. Additionally, you may be able to use your insurance to help with the expenses. Check each site for more details.

BetterHelp : https://www.betterhelp.com/get-started/
This site provides therapy resources for individuals, couples, and teens. Therapists are assigned based on a short questionnaire. **BetterHelp** offers a variety of ways to reach your therapist for appointments and assistance.

TalkSpace : https://try.talkspace.com/
This site allows users to custom-tailor their program to their current

needs. TalkSpace also includes medication management services for those who are interested in assistance with their medication.

Wellnite : https://www.wellnite.com/
This site connects with several insurance plans and provides both therapy and medication management services. Appointments are available for individuals, teens, families, and couples.

Amwell : https://patients.amwell.com/conditions/depression/
This site provides online assistance for a variety of medical conditions, including mental illnesses such as depression, anxiety, and OCD. They also offer night, weekend, and holiday sessions based on availability and need.

Teladoc : https://www.teladochealth.com/
This site provides virtual medical care for a variety of situations and conditions. You may wish to check with your employer or insurance coverage to determine if your use of Teladoc is covered under your plan.

Pride Counseling : https://www.pridecounseling.com/faq/
This resource provides specialized care for those who identify as part of the LGBTQIA+ community.

Faithful Counseling : https://www.faithfulcounseling.com/faq/
This site provides faith-based Christian counseling services for those who are struggling with mental health issues.

Ayana Therapy : https://www.ayanatherapy.com/

This resource provides care for members of the BIPOC community with an interest providing culturally appropriate counseling for everyone.

Regain : https://www.regain.us/faq/

This site focuses on couples and partner therapy. Mental health and emotional management can be a team effort for committed couples, and Regain provides services for each partner in addition to couples care.

What You Should Know :

https://www.apa.org/topics/telehealth/online-therapy

If this is your first time trying online therapy, the American Psychological Association has provided this fantastic guide to things you should keep in mind when weighing the pros and cons of each potential service.

Articles and Associated Psychology Websites

There are seemingly endless articles regarding the interplay between mental and emotional health. Typing in a term like "emotional and mental health" into a search engine can return a seemingly bottomless pit of articles, ranging from highly scientific to spiritual to mystical to deeply opinionated.

If you are interested in researching your mental health diagnoses or status, I urge you to use equal doses of good sense and caution. You may encounter sites that claim you can "cure yourself" of mental illness through a specific process invented by someone who may or may not be affiliated with the medical or psychological community. I am personally of the opinion that methods which do not cause harm to you or others and that provide you with relief, confidence, mindfulness tools, and a deeper understanding of who you are, psychologically and emotionally speaking, are all equally good options. Things like crystals, sound baths, aromatherapy, CBD, and yoga are often criticized for not passing the test of peer-reviewed, medically investigated proof of relief. However, the same could be said of a teddy bear or comfort blanket. If you believe that what you are doing is helping you find balance and serenity, and it is not a threat to you, your livelihood, or those around you, then I see no reason to not enjoy yourself. I also see no reason in starting arguments because of conflicting opinions about the validity of these methods.

Therefore, in collecting these articles from around the internet, I tried to find a variety that would appeal to a diverse audience. I have provided a brief description of each article, so that you may choose only those which personally interest you.

Is There a Difference Between Emotional Health and Mental Health? :https://www.redoakrecovery.com/addiction-blog/emotional-health-vs-mental-health/
This entry is part of an addiction recovery center's blog but should not be misconstrued as an endorsement– I have no affiliation with this business, but they have a great blog!

Mood instability is a common feature of mental health disorders and is associated with poor clinical outcomes : https://www.ncbi.nlm.nih.gov/pmc/articles/PMC4452754/
The National Library of Medicine is a fantastic resource for those interested in current research regarding mental illnesses and the overlap between

mental health and emotional health. Instead of articles, this site provides published scientific studies.

Mental Illness and The Importance of Stability :
https://www.healthyplace.com/other-info/mental-health-newsletter/mental-illness-and-the-importance-of-stability
HealthyPlace has a wealth of resources pertaining to mental and emotional health. Each article is presented in familiar terms and includes helpful links that have the potential to lead anyone down a rabbit hole of fascinating scientific and personal discussions of mental health issues.

Addressing Emotions with Mental Illness:
https://www.nami.org/Blogs/NAMI-Blog/May-2020/Addressing-Emotions-with-Mental-Illness
The National Alliance on Mental Illness (NAMI) is another thorough resource. Articles here are a bit more on the scientific side but are presented cohesively. NAMI provides specialized information for a variety of cultures and communities as well as resources for professionals.

Mental Illness and the Family: Recognizing Warning Signs and How to Cope :
https://www.mhanational.org/recognizing-warning-signs
Mental Health America– MHA– is a nonprofit organization providing mental health care assistance through advocacy, education, and local resources.

For more information on finding help through MHA :
https://www.mhanational.org/finding-help

5 Ways Almost Everyone Misunderstands Emotions :
https://www.psychologytoday.com/us/blog/in-prac-
tice/202207/5-ways-almost-everyone-misunderstands-emo-
tions?amp

Psychology Today magazine was founded in 1967, and since then has become the world's largest portal to mental health and behavioral science resources. Articles vary in length and scientific language, and can connect readers with a variety of schools of thought and theories.

Social Media Outlets, Forums, Groups, and Pages

The internet is both wonderful and terrible for people struggling with mental illness and emotional issues. On one hand, we have the opportunity to connect with other individuals who understand what we're going through. On the other hand, many online portals with open comment sections can be an outlet for people to spew misinformation and hateful opinions. Additionally, it can become very easy to engage with social media and forums to an unhealthy extent.

Therefore, I've provided a few options that could be helpful, but I recommend proceeding with caution. There may be mention of triggering topics and unfriendly comments. However, if you are in a place where you can laugh and empathize with others regarding mutual circumstances, these can be a helpful resource for restoring a little mindfulness to your day.

Illustrated Instagram Accounts:
The Latest Kate : Original animal-based artwork celebrating mindful-ness and positivity.

Marcela Ilustra : Marcela is a Brazilian artist who creates drawings that illustrate mental health struggles and the logical reality of these situations that we often miss.

Sarah Andersen : This comic focuses on some of the humorous and ridiculous aspects of trying to maintain mental health.

Chuck Draws Things : This comic features a flock of pigeons and their relatable coping mechanisms.

Real Depression Project : Provides quotes and content provided by others along with narratives to help individuals and their support team better understand the scope of mental illness.

Facebook Pages:

The You Rock Foundation Facebook Page : A nonprofit organization that raises awareness for suicide prevention through music.

Mental Health Awareness Life Facebook Page : Their mission statement says it all: "dedicated to raising awareness, inspiration, education, and support around: mental health, mental wellness, mental illnesses, and personal development."

Multiple Resource Websites:

Depression Army : With a focus on depression, this page helps de-stigmatize mental illness. (depressionarmy.com)

The Mighty : A community-based approach to living with a variety of wellness issues including mental health concerns.
(themighty.com)

Stigma Fighters : This site allows individuals to submit their own unique story and read those of others who live with mental illness.
(stigmafighters.com)

Online Apps

In our technology-focused world, apps have become a popular way to practice mindfulness and unwind. Apps can be very beneficial because they are portable— you can access them from your mobile phone or tablet, making assistance as close as your pocket.

There are dozens of apps available in each category, so consider this just a place to get started in your search for apps that can benefit you. While most apps are available for all operating systems, you may wish to double-check which are available for Apple versus Android devices. Additionally, there may be a cost associated with some apps.

Some apps might not be right for you, while others are a perfect fit, so take your time researching and investigating before you commit to any app.

Journal Apps
Daylio : https://daylio.net/
Longwalks : https://longwalks.com/
Reflectly : https://reflectly.app/
Zinnia Journal and Planner : https://www.pixiteapps.com/apps/zinnia-digital-journaling-app/
Reflect Guided Daily Journal : https://www.reflectjournal.com/

Mindfulness Apps
Headspace : https://www.headspace.com/headspace-meditation-app
Calm : https://www.calm.com/

Mindfulness Coach : https://mobile.va.gov/app/mindfulness-coach
Anxiety Solution : https://www.anxietysolution.app/
Buddhify : https://buddhify.com/

Cognitive Behavior Therapy
MoodKit : https://www.thriveport.com/products/moodkit/
MindShift : https://www.anxietycanada.com/resources/mindshift-cbt/
Bloom : https://bloombetteryou.com/
Sanvello : https://www.sanvello.com/
MoodMission : https://moodmission.com/

Exercises, Techniques, and More Information

These resources include workbooks, therapy guides, and other tools gathered by professionals in the mental health field. In some cases, these materials are used as part of therapy sessions, and have been chosen because they have the potential to provide guidance to different individuals. You may wish to review each resource with your professional care team before implementing the ideas and exercises addressed in each one to ensure it's a good fit for you, your current mental status, and your overall goals.

Individual Therapy Manual for Cognitive-Behavioral Treatment of Depression by Ricardo F. Munoz and Jeanne Miranda (PDF)

A Course in CBT Techniques: A Free Online CBT Workbook by Albert Bonfil, PsyD and Suraji Wagage PhD, JD (web-based)

5 Surprisingly Effective Cognitive Behavioral Therapy Exercises by Dr. Konstantin Lukin

This article is presented in conjunction with Dr. Lukin's own practice and includes video content from the provider.

Psychology Tools for Living Well
This is an online self-help course that provides users with reading material and exercises to help them improve their mental health and lifestyle.

Think CBT Wheel of Emotions
Think CBT provides a variety of worksheets to help providers and patients alike understand and practice skills learned through therapy. This Wheel of Emotions can be useful for helping you identify how you feel when things get rough.

Topic Ideas and Prompts

Earlier in this book, we discussed how prompts can help us get into the groove of journaling and even mindfulness. There are several ways you can use the following prompts:

- As topic ideas for your journal entries
- As a focus for meditation
- As something to contemplate through the day
- As a discussion topic for your support team or community
- As inspiration for your next creative endeavor

The following 25 prompts cover a variety of concepts, topics, ideas, and emotions, so it may be helpful to read through them when you are having a hard time processing your thoughts.

Whether or not you deeply ponder or journal about these topics, it can also be helpful to pause and reflect on them for a moment or two, especially when you're feeling lots of stress or experiencing a myriad of emotions simultaneously. You may wish to refer to this list for inspiration as well.

- How do you show compassion to those around you? What would it take to give yourself that same compassion?

- List three things you'd like to tell a friend, family member, or partner.

- What values do you consider most important in life (honesty, integrity, loyalty, sense of humor, etc.)? How do you demonstrate these values? What kind of changes could you make to make these values more prominent?

- Describe yourself using just ten words or traits. Consider if there are any traits you wish could describe you and brainstorm how you might be able to develop those traits.

- What is your favorite thing about yourself? What attributes trouble you?

- Finish this sentence: "My life would not be the same without ..."

- Describe a time when you trusted yourself. How hard is it for you to trust your own instincts and logic?

- What are three things you wish everybody knew or under-stood about you?

- What negative thoughts or difficult emotions do you experience most regularly? Are you experiencing them now?

- Which emotions do you find hardest to accept (guilt, anger, sadness, etc.)? What do you feel like when these emotions present themselves to you?

- Describe a choice you regret. Now describe what you learned from that experience that has improved your life since the event.

- What parts of daily life cause the most emotional stress? What can you do to change those experiences or situations?

- Identify three trigger scenarios in which something can quickly bring about negative emotions and self-talk. What strategies do you currently use when these things happen?

- What are your top three negative thoughts about yourself? What would these thoughts look like if you were to reframe them through positivity?

- What are your immediate coping strategies to help you get through moments of emotional duress?

- Who do you trust when you are experiencing emotional pain or psychological distress? How can you connect with them when you're feeling less than ideal?

- What is your greatest fear? How has this changed throughout your life?

- What words have impacted your life and molded how you think about something?

- What are five things that would make me feel fulfilled? How can I incorporate them into my life?

- When do you feel the most scared?

- Describe a time you felt your absolute best. What was it about that moment that was so amazing? How do you think you could capture this sensation again?

- What's something you wish you had known in your younger years? How would things be different if you knew then what you know now? How can you apply what you've learned to your current and future self?

- What are you doing today that will benefit you tomorrow?

- How do you handle conflicts and disagreements? What changes would you like to make to this method?

- What do you need to do to feel balanced and ready to face the world?

Printed in Great Britain
by Amazon

86759523R00072